Voices of Scleroderma
Volume 2

Voices of Scleroderma
Volume 2

Editors
Judith Thompson Devlin & Shelley L. Ensz
for the
International Scleroderma Network

ISN Press

Voices of Scleroderma Volume 2, First Edition

Editors Judith Thompson Devlin and Shelley L. Ensz
Senior Editors Sonya Detwiler and Maia Dock
Production Saba Sadiq
Cover Art Ione Bridgman
Cover Art Assistant Sherrill Knaggs
Distribution Christine Patane

Published by ISN Press7455 France Avenue South, #266, Edina, MN 55435.

Printed and bound in the United States of America.

Disclaimer: We do not endorse or recommend any treatment for scleroderma or related illnesses. Please consult your doctor or scleroderma expert for treatment advice.

Sources: All personal stories in this book were originally published on the ww.sclero.org website and are reprinted here with written permission of the authors. Pen names have been used when requested and in many instances, author names are different between the website and book stories. All stories have been edited for clarity and content for this book.

Library of Congress Control Number: 2004105617
Publisher: BookSurge, LLC
North Charleston, South Carolina

ISBN: 0-9724623-1-7

Dedication

Lives of great men all remind us
We can make our lives sublime,
And, departing, leave behind us
Footprints on the sands of time.

Footprints, that perhaps another,
Sailing o'er life's solemn main,
A forlorn and shipwrecked brother,
Seeing, shall take heart again.

— Henry Wadsworth Longfellow
From "A Psalm of Life"

To all the great people herein who have helped others
take heart again by letting their voice be heard
in the worldwide fight against scleroderma,
"the disease that turns people to stone."

Table of Contents

Part 1: Systemic Scleroderma

Chapter 1: Systemic Scleroderma Medical Information

Scleroderma Related Pulmonary Hypertension
by Carol M. Black, MD, FRCP, CBE
and Christopher P. Denton, PhD, FRCP

Molière, Maurice Raynaud and Modern Measures of Microcirculation
Introduction to Scleroderma Fibroblasts

Chapter 2: Systemic Scleroderma Caregiver Stories

Chapter 3: Systemic Scleroderma Patient Stories

Part 2: Juvenile and Localized Scleroderma

Chapter 5: Juvenile Scleroderma

Medical Overview of Juvenile Scleroderma (JSD)

Juvenile Scleroderma

Chapter 6: Localized Scleroderma (Linear and Morphea)

Part 3: Autoimmune and Overlap

Chapter 7: Autoimmune Stories

Chapter 8: Overlap, UCTD and MCTD Stories

Part 4: International

Chapter 9: Español (Spanish)

Chapter 10: Italiano (Italian)

Chapter 11: Polski (Polish)

Chapter 12: Русский (Russian)

◆❖◆

Acknowledgments
by Judith Thompson Devlin and Shelley L. Ensz

Judith Thompson Devlin is Chair of the Archivist Committee for the International Scleroderma Network (ISN). Shelley Ensz is Founder and President of the International Scleroderma Network, the ISN's Scleroderma from A to Z Web site at www.sclero.org, and the Scleroderma Webmaster's Association.

This book features over one hundred stories and was created by over one hundred and fifty global volunteers who have worked together via the Internet, cutting across all the barriers of language and politics to share information and support with each other.

All the proceeds of this book series will benefit the nonprofit patient organization, the International Scleroderma Network (ISN).

Certainly, the first credit for this book goes to everyone who has shared their story on ISN's *Scleroderma from A to Z* website where these stories were first posted and where the inspiration for this book was born. These stories are the heart, the soul, and the lifeblood of the website where we all first met and the international nonprofit that we became.

Many thanks go to Arnold Slotkin, a dear friend who calmly insisted that forming the ISN nonprofit would be a fitting outgrowth of the website, despite Shelley's many objections. He gracefully weathered many emails spouting, "Arnold, this is all your fault!" But, of course, it is really to his everlasting credit.

Shelley also extends hearty thanks to Judith, for this book and series would not have existed without her enthusiastic urging and leadership. Judith generously volunteered to archive this series the day after the ISN was publicly launched on January 21, 2002.

ISN board members who were more heavily involved with this book series include Gene Ensz, Joanne Grow, and Nolan LaTourelle. Linda K. Hopkins of Intelliware International Law Firm, who is Chair of the ISN Legal Advisory Council, provided invaluable advice for this series.

Ione Bridgman, who is an ISN Artist, painted our beautiful cover design to illustrate this book's theme of offering hope, with the lighthouse and rainbow. Sherrill Knaggs created the digital art from Ione's painting.

Senior editors for this book included Sonya Detwiler and Maia Dock. We are enormously grateful for their wisdom, skill and persistence in polishing this manuscript.

Saba Sadiq handled the prepress for this volume, which entailed layout, typography, and design. She also serves as Assistant Webmaster for our website.

Christine Patane, who is ISN Membership and Donation Coordinator, did the final verification of mailing addresses for this book series and prepared the shipping labels for the first edition books which were signed and sent by Judith Thompson Devlin.

The ISN Medical Advisory Board is led by Dr. James Seibold, who has written the Introduction to this volume. He is Professor of Internal Medicine and Director of the University of Michigan Scleroderma Program in Ann Arbor, Michigan. Author of more than three hundred scientific publications, he is considered a world thought leader in scleroderma, Raynaud's phenomenon, and interventional research in the rheumatologic diseases.

Professional contributors to this volume include Professor Carol Black, Dr. Christopher Denton, Kevin Howell, Dr. Vanessa Malcarne, Dr. L Nandini Moorthy, and Dr. Maria Trojanowska.

We are very thankful for Professor Black and Dr. Christopher Denton's article on pulmonary hypertension, which is the medical centerpiece of this volume.

Professor Carol Black, MD, FRCP, CBE, is the Director of the Department of Rheumatology at Royal Free Hospital in London, England, and a renowned expert in scleroderma. The department has an active research program. For her lifetime work she was honored with the prestigious award of Commander of the British Empire (CBE). Professor Black is also President of the Royal College of Physicians in London.

Dr. Christopher Denton, PhD, FRCP, is Senior Lecturer and Consultant Rheumatologist at the Scleroderma Clinic, Centre for Rheumatology of Royal Free Hospital. He has more than ten years of experience dealing with scleroderma and related disorders. He completed a PhD in Vascular Biology in 1997 and then trained for two years in molecular genetics in Houston before taking up his faculty position in Professor Black's unit at Royal Free.

Kevin Howell contributed a wonderful article about Raynaud's and microcirculation. He is a Clinical Scientist for Professor Black at the Royal Free Hospital in London. He began working in the field of scleroderma in 1991, and uses the techniques of capillaroscopy and infrared thermography.

Dr. Vanessa Malcarne has written a very compelling article, "Developing Empathy: A Researcher's Perspective on Being Diagnosed with Scleroderma." She is Professor, Department of Psychology at San Diego State University. Her research focuses on quality of life for people with cancer and rheumatic diseases (including scleroderma). She also studies the effects of chronic illness on spouses and children.

Dr. L. Nandini Moorthy wrote the introduction for our juvenile scleroderma chapter. She is Assistant Professor of Pediatric Rheumatology at UMDNJ/Robert Wood Johnson Medical School in New Brunswick, New Jersey.

Dr. Maria Trojanowska is Associate Professor, Division of Rheumatology and Immunology at the Medical University of South Carolina. The main area of research in her laboratory is regulation of extracellular matrix (ECM) deposition in healthy tissues and its dysregulation in diseases. Her article on scleroderma fibroblasts nicely explains the importance of these specialized cells that are responsible for making connective tissue. She dedicates her article to the memory of Dr. E. Carwile LeRoy, who was one of the pioneers in scleroderma research, and he was well known and admired around the world.

All stories in this book are printed in their original language as well as translated into English. Translators for stories that appear in this book include Dr. Magdalena Dziadzio, Kevin Howell, Dr. Roy Smith, Edwin Lamoli-Torres, and Dr. Alexandra Balbir-Gurman. Additionally, dozens of other translators are involved in the preparation and maintenance of our multilingual website.

Dr. Magdalena Dziadzio has served in many capacities with the ISN over the past three years. She is the lead author of several abstracts presented at EULAR (the European League Against Rheumatism) Conferences in 2003 and 2004, based on analysis of our ISN website inquiries, entitled, *Internet as a Tool for Patient Support Groups to Provide Quality Information.*

She also arranged for many of the professional articles in this book series, and translated stories and related emails for us for several different languages. Dr. Dziadzio developed her knowledge about scleroderma working with Professor Carol Black and her team at the Department of Rheumatology at Royal Free Hospital in London, where she is currently working on a research project.

Dr. Roy Smith graduated from the University of Cambridge, England, with a degree in Natural Sciences. He has been working in the field of Medical Electronics. He collaborates with the Royal Free Hospital's Department of Rheumatology, led by Professor Carol Black, in the area of physiological measurements such as thermography and laser Doppler flowmetry.

Edwin Lamoli-Torres is a retired professor from the University of Puerto Rico at Mayaguez. Edwin received his Master's Degree in ESL from Teacher's College, Columbia University in New York City.

Dr. Alexandra Balbir-Gurman is a Senior Rheumatologist at Rambam Medical Center in Haifa, Israel. She graduated from the Chernovits School of Medicine in the former USSR (Ukraine). In 2000, she did six months of training and clinical work under the supervision of Professor Carol Black at Royal Free Hospital.

Finally, this book was published with generous funding from an anonymous donor, in loving memory of Marta Marx, who will always be remembered as a truly outstanding benefactress to scleroderma research.

Please keep in mind that scleroderma affects everyone differently. There is no predictable course for any form of the disease. Nothing in this book is intended as personal medical advice, so please consult your doctor before making any changes to lifestyle or treatments. We do our best to keep the most current information on treatments and clinical trials available on our website.

With so many people involved in this book's production, the only thing for certain is that there are countless people who have played a vital role in its success who are not mentioned here. Many of them are profiled on our website as ISN Representatives or supporters. Some of our volunteers prefer to work anonymously or behind the scenes. Their names deserve to be here also, and they are woven throughout this book in spirit.

We hope it will suffice to say that if you have ever helped the cause of scleroderma in any way, anywhere in the world, you have done a great and grand deed, and we are all very thankful for your footprints in the sand.

◆ ❖ ◆

Introduction
by James R. Seibold, M.D.

Dr. Seibold is Chair of the ISN Medical Advisory Board. He is Professor of Internal Medicine and Director of the University of Michigan Scleroderma Program in Ann Arbor, Michigan, USA.

We welcome you to *Voices of Scleroderma*, a major contribution from the International Scleroderma Network (ISN).

Scleroderma occurs in only around thirty people per million per year. Therefore, since it is so uncommon, patients have great difficulty finding access to expert care or even another similarly afflicted patient with whom they can share their experience.

Access to high quality reliable modern information is crucial to patient well-being and outcomes. The realization that "you ARE NOT alone" has therapeutic value in its own right.

I am Chair of the ISN Medical Advisory, a scleroderma researcher, and a member of the Scleroderma Clinical Trials Consortium. The SCTC is an international charitable organization of academic centers dedicated to elevating the pace and quality of scleroderma research. The SCTC works closely with the ISN in the education of both patients and caregivers.

I have been interacting with the ISN on a variety of fronts, most notably in our shared goal of providing up to date and accurate information to the scleroderma community on a worldwide basis. Over the past six years, I have watched the amazing development of the site that Shelley Ensz created at www.sclero.org. I have seen it evolve from her personal site of one page to become the ISN site, now encompassing over one thousand pages in eighteen languages.

The ISN site has brought together both the medical and patient communities from throughout the world. According to the recent TrustGauge Report of Internet traffic, it is in the top one hundred thousand of all Web sites, far ahead of all other scleroderma-related sites.

In my view, the primary reason for this stellar success is the high quality of site content, as well as the multilingual, international reach, which is also an important driving force. Remarkably, the ISN has a small team of committed, dedicated volunteers who have seized the amazing capabilities of the Internet to provide exceptional, worldwide service and assistance to patients with scleroderma.

More notably, from this enterprising site, the ISN has in turn developed into a thriving nonprofit organization. It is really a classic example of reversing the order of development. Rather than an established organization simply developing a Web site, a remarkably effective Web site developed into a full-service charitable organization.

The ISN expands upon its cyberspace outreach by publishing *Voices of Scleroderma*. Every volume in this book series features articles from esteemed scleroderma researchers as well as over one hundred patient and caregiver stories, from sixteen countries, and in five languages.

The ISN enjoys a well-deserved reputation for top-notch medical and support information and services from both the patient and medical organizations throughout the world. Today, over five dozen dedicated volunteers, including many doctors and translators, operate the ISN.

Our ISN Medical Advisory Board includes illustrious experts in this field, such as Dr. Luis Catoggio of Buenos Aires, Argentina; Dr. Marco Mattucci-Cerinic of Florence, Italy; Dr. C. Stephen Foster of Boston, Massachusetts; Dr. Janet Pope of London, Ontario; Dr. Frank van den Hoogen of The Netherlands; and Dr. Shinichi Sato of Kanazawa, Japan.

Dozens of other renowned leaders in their field also generously lend their expertise to the ISN, primarily as contributing authors, medical editors, scientific advisors, and translators.

All of our ISN volunteers met and work only through the Internet. Their efforts have made quality medical and support information on this rare disease available worldwide.

I hope you find this book of value, and that you also consider offering support to the ISN. It is only with a partnership of patients and scientists in a concerted worldwide effort that we will solve the riddle of scleroderma.

◆ ❖ ◆

PART 1

Systemic Scleroderma

CHAPTER 1

Systemic Scleroderma
Medical Information

*Fortunately there have been major
clinical advances in the management of
pulmonary hypertension over the past five years.*
—Professor Carol M. Black

Scleroderma Related Pulmonary Hypertension
by Carol M. Black, MD, FRCP, CBE
and Christopher P. Denton, PhD, FRCP

Professor Carol Black is the Director of the Department of Rheumatology at Royal Free Hospital in London, England, and a renowned expert in scleroderma. She is also President of the Royal College of Physicians in London, UK.

Dr. Chris Denton is Senior Lecturer and Consultant Rheumatologist for the Scleroderma Clinic, Centre for Rheumatology at Royal Free Hospital.

Introduction

Pulmonary arterial hypertension is a common complication of systemic sclerosis, although the exact prevalence is unclear. However, in most hospital based series it is around 10 to 15%[1]. Pulmonary arterial hypertension (PAH) is not all of one type in systemic sclerosis (SSc).

First there are cases, especially complicating limited cutaneous systemic sclerosis (lcSSc), in which there is severe isolated pulmonary arterial hypertension.

Secondly there are cases of PAH complicating severe interstitial pulmonary fibrosis and which is associated with hypoxia, and thirdly there may be another type of pulmonary vascular disease occurring in SSc that reflects the general vascular pathology of the disease and results in a more indolent pulmonary process. These are individuals who have a secondary pulmonary vascular component in the context of relatively mild fibrosis, distinct from the severe interstitial process seen in true secondary PAH and those who appear to have very slowly progressive PAH in the context of limited cutaneous systemic sclerosis (lcSSc).

Thus, although there are similarities between idiopathic or familial primary PAH and SSc-associated isolated PAH, these do not apply to all cases. Drawing analogy with other aspects of the disease clinical heterogeneity seems likely and it may ultimately be possible to subclassify this complication just as the patterns of lung fibrosis, skin involvement or severity of Raynaud's phenomenon may be segregated.

The earliest reports of pulmonary arterial hypertension as a complication of scleroderma are of historical interest[2, 3], but it has almost certainly been an under recognised complication and may well have often been misdiagnosed as interstitial pulmonary fibrosis, asthma or as heart failure of unknown cause. It is likely that cases of cardiac involvement from SSc are in some cases attributable to decompensated pulmonary arterial hypertension.

There has been an excess of cardiac mortality in almost all series of SSc survival published and a substantial proportion of deaths may have resulted from unrecognised pulmonary vascular disease or secondary cardiac problems.

Fortunately there have been major clinical advances in the management of PAH over the past five years. In particular there have now been several clinical trials confirming efficacy for parenteral or inhaled prostacyclin analogues and also for an oral endothelin receptor antagonist—these therapies are now licensed in many countries for use in primary or connective tissue disease associated PAH.

Prevalence

The prevalence of PAH in scleroderma is difficult to determine. There is a wide range in reported series. This probably results from differences in diagnostic criteria and patient populations examined. The best data come from cardiac catheter studies, although this may underdiagnose as most patients must raise clinical suspicion of PAH in order to proceed to this invasive test. Our own data suggest a prevalence of 12 to 15% in a hospital-based cohort. This is within the published range of 5 to 50% of SSc cases[4].

The relationship between the severity or pattern of SSc and PAH is unclear. The isolated form is associated with classical lcSSc (previously termed CREST syndrome) and with ACA reactivity. It is also seen in dcSSc associated with anti fibrillarin autoantibodies (U3RNP). When scleroderma overlaps with other diseases such as the antiphospholipid antibody syndrome or systemic lupus erythematosus (SLE), other mechanisms may be operating.

Survival

PAH in SSc has a major impact on quality of life, survival and outcome. A pivotal study by Koh et al studied a small number of cases of scleroderma related PAH and determined a median survival of 12 months. Here PAH diagnosis was based upon echocardiography. A study from our own unit suggested differences in survival according to the level of PAH by echo-Doppler at diagnosis. Thus for PAH above 30 mmHg survival was 20% at 20 months[5]. These simple studies probably overlook important differences between SSc-PAH patients. As discussed earlier it is likely that different patterns of disease have varying natural histories and this may reflect fundamental differences between patient subsets and/or pathogenic process. It is however clear that advanced PAH is progressive and has a high mortality. It is less clear how milder forms progress and whether the difference in natural history suggested by cohort studies reflects earlier diagnosis or different progression. This is an important question for future examination.

Clinical aspects

The clinical classification of pulmonary hypertension is complex (**Table 1**). Most cases of SSc related pulmonary hypertension are within the Pulmonary Arterial Hypertension subset, although occasionally Chronic Obstructive Airways Disease (COPD) and associated sarcoidosis is the cause (**Table 1**). Current criteria define PAH as a resting mean PAP above 25mm Hg or an exercise mean PAP of greater than 30 mm Hg. These levels are accepted internationally and such standardisation is vital for comparison of cohorts and standardisation of therapy.

Clinical features can be misleading and probably occur relatively late in the natural history of the disease. The earliest symptom is usually exertional breathlessness or reduced exercise capacity. Symptomatically this leads to dyspnoea on exertion and commonly patients notice this when climbing stairs or hills. Later this dyspnoea occurs at rest.

Scleroderma patients may be dyspnoeic for other reasons—anaemia, interstitial pulmonary disease or mechanical restriction in ventilation, muscloskeletal disease, or exercise tolerance, and these must be excluded. Other symptoms that occur at later stages are chest pain due to right ventricular angina and syncope or near syncope on exertion due to reduced cardiac reserve.

Late-stage disease leads to features of right-sided cardiac failure, including ankle swelling. Operationally PAH can be graded into fours groups based upon modified New York Heart Association criteria. The widely used Class I to IV classification is summarised in **Table 2**.

In early disease the clinical features can be unrewarding, but in established disease clinical examination can be confirmatory with features of a loud pulmonary second sound due to accelerated valve closure, parasternal heave due to right ventricular strain and signs of elevated right sided filling pressures (elevated JVP and prominent jugular venous pulsation, together with fluid retention (ankle/sacral oedema, ascites).

Table 1: World Health Organisation Diagnostic Classification of Pulmonary Hypertension (1998)

1. Pulmonary Arterial Hypertension
   1.1   Primary Pulmonary Hypertension
         (a) Sporadic
         (b) Familial
   1.2   Related to:
         (a) Connective tissue disease
         (b) Congenital Systemic to Pulmonary Shunts
         (c) Portal Hypertension
         (d) HIV Infection
         (e) Drugs/Toxins
             (1) Anorexigens
             (2) Other
         (f) Persistent Pulmonary Hypertension of the Newborn
         (g) Other

2. Pulmonary Venous Hypertension
   2.1   Left-Sided Atrial or Ventricular Heart Disease
   2.2   Left-Sided Valvular Heart Disease
   2.3   Extrinsic Compression of Central Pulmonary Veins
         (a) Fibrosing Mediastinitis
         (b) Adenopathy/Tumors
   2.4   Pulmonary Veno-Occlusive disease
   2.5   Other

3. Pulmonary Hypertension Associated with Disorders of the Respiratory System and/or Hypoxemia
   3.1   Chronic Obstructive Pulmonary Disease (COPD)
   3.2   Interstitial Lung Disease
   3.3   Sleep Disordered Breathing
   3.4   Alveolar Hypoventilation Disorders
   3.5   Chronic Exposure to High Altitude
   3.6   Neonatal Lung Disease
   3.7   Alveolar-Capillary Dysplasia
   3.8   Other

4. Pulmonary Hypertension due to Chronic Thrombotic and/or Embolic Disease
   4.1   Thromboembolic Obstruction of Proximal Pulmonary Arteries
   4.2   Obstruction of Distal Pulmonary Arteries
         (a) Pulmonary Embolism (Thrombus, Tumour, Ova/parasites, foreign material)
         (b) In-situ Thrombosis
         (c) Sickle Cell Disease

5. Pulmonary Hypertension due to Disorders Directly Affecting the Pulmonary Vasculature
   5.1   Infammatory
         (a) Schistosomiasis
         (b) Sarcoidosis
         (c) Other
   5.2   Pulmonary Capillary Haemangiomatosis

Late events are tachypnoea at rest or central cyanosis. Anecdotal evidence suggests that patients with significant isolated PAH in lcSSc often have extensive and increasing cutaneous vascular lesions.

Preclinical or early diagnosis cannot depend on clinical features. Routine repeated investigations are the correct way in which to manage a patient. Traditionally in systemic sclerosis most emphasis has been placed upon a combination of PFT and Doppler-echocardiography[6]. ECG should not be relied upon as changes are often late and likely to be present on Echo before the ECG becomes abnormal.

The most typical PFT abnormality in isolated PAH is a reduction in CO transfer factor (Tlco) with preservation of lung volumes. The Dlco appears to be less subject to variation than the Kco, although this is generally proportionately reduced in these cases. However isolated and often transient changes in CO diffusing capacity are quite common in SSc. The explanation for this is unclear but may relate to altered regulation of ventilation and perfusion resulting in V:Q mismatch.

Pulmonary function tests therefore must be interpreted in the clinical context of which a patient's change in symptoms are an important contributor and repeated if results seem inconsistent. Tobacco smoking will also lead to a depressed transfer factor.

Echocardiography has been shown to be a useful tool for PAH assessment. Accuracy of the measurement varies, assessment is operator dependent and a mild degree of regurgitation may be especially hard to assess.

Doppler-echocardiography is most reliable when performed by an experienced observer. In this case it has a high sensitivity and specificity [7] for detecting PAH. Observations of importance are an increased pulmonary acceleration time, altered movement of the interventricular septum and impaired right ventricular function or pulmonary outflow dilatation.

It is also possible to estimate the peak (systolic) pulmonary artery pressure by combining echocardiography with Doppler assessment of the regurgitant blood jet velocity through the tricuspid valve. Overall there is a good correlation between Doppler estimated peak PAP and that determined at right heart catheter, but in practice this is influenced by extreme values and in the clinically important range of 30 to 45mm peak pressure has false positive or negative rates of around 30%.

Attempts to improve diagnostic sensitivity are being assessed. Most promising are stress tests, especially performing echo assessment during or immediately after exercise. The former requires specialised equipment but has produced promising data[8], the latter has only been used so far in small studies but may be useful. Dopamine stress testing so far does not appear to be especially additive to regular tests.

Right heart catheterisation

This is the gold standard for investigation of PAH in all contexts. The advantages of right heart catheterisation (RHC) include the direct measurement of PAP, determination of mean PAP which is used for defining true PAH, and ability to perform a stress test to identify exercise induced PAH that might not be measurable at rest.

Vasodilator challenge can also be performed to assess pulmonary vascular responsiveness. In SSc-PAH this is rarely positive. Scleroderma patients are rarely responsive to oral vasodilators such as Nifedipene and the result of the test does not appear to associate with outcome.

In PPH it has been suggested that responsive patients might benefit from high dose vasodilator therapy with calcium channel blockers, although this is controversial. RHC also allows accurate measurement of cardiac index, a measure of cardiac output corrected for body size, pulmonary vascular resistance and other indices. These appear to have important prognostic value when related to outcome or survival.

Table 2: 1998 World Health Organisation Functional Classification of Pulmonary Hypertension (Modified after the New York Heart Association Functional Classification)

Class I   Patients with pulmonary hypertension but without resulting limitation of physical activity. Ordinary physical activity does not cause undue dyspnoea or fatigue, chest pain or near syncope.

Class II   Patients with pulmonary hypertension resulting in slight limitation of physical activity. They are comfortable at rest. Ordinary physical activity causes undue dyspnoea, fatigue, chest pain or near syncope.

Class III   Patients with pulmonary hypertension resulting in marked limitation of physical activity. They are comfortable at rest. Ordinary physical activity causes undue dyspnoea or fatigue, chest pain or near syncope.

Class IV   Patients with pulmonary hypertension with inability to carry out any physical activity without symptoms. These patients manifest signs of right heart failure. Dyspnoea and/or fatigue may even be present at rest. Discomfort is increased by any physical activity.

Currently in the UK it is regarded as mandatory to have RHC information in order to commence advanced PAH therapy.[9] In situations where coexistent left ventricular disease is suspected it may be useful to perform a left heart catheter and coronary angiogram at the same time as the RHC. Should thromboembolic disease be suspected then a V:Q Scan or CT-pulmonary angiogram should be performed. The range of investigations central to accurate assessment of PAH in SSc are listed in **Table 3**.

Monitoring

Monitoring of all patients with SSc by annual Doppler-echocardiogram is recommended by the World Health Organization (WHO), and *concomitant* pulmonary function testing is now accepted as the standard of practice in Europe and North America.

Once the diagnosis has been made it is important that it is followed and this is probably most practically done by serial Doppler-echocardiography every 3 to 6 months depending upon clinical change and also by symptom severity and exercise capacity. The 6MWT has been established as a reproducible simple clinical measure of exercise capacity in PAH and this associates with progression and survival. It should be regularly performed in all patients using a marked 50m course. There are defined levels of encouragement and patients decide when the test is complete unless they exceed 500m. Some centres perform arterial desaturation tests using arterialised earlobe blood sampling or pulse oximetry. This may be misleading in SSc due to coexistent Raynaud's phenomenon.

Differential diagnosis and classification

There are now well-established WHO diagnostic criteria for PAH.[9] Clinical features and investigations such as ECG, Doppler-echocardiogram and pulmonary function tests are useful and also assist with important differential diagnoses such as cardiac involvement or interstitial lung fibrosis. Thromboembolic disease must be excluded and V:Q scans or CTPA are important.

Additional cardiac tests might also be needed to exclude coronary arterial or intrinsic cardiac disease and inflammatory myocarditis must be considered in relevant cases. This condition is often associated with elevated CKMB and troponin levels. Gated cardiac MRI appears to be a valuable research tool that may be applied to the diagnosis of both cardiac and pulmonary vascular disease through its effects on cardiac cavity and muscle mass and movement.

Aetiopathogenesis

The aetiology of PAH in SSc is likely to be complex and multifactorial. The initial event is unclear but a possible sequence of events involves a predisposed individual, including genetic predispositions that are likely to be a result of a balance between protective or predisposing alleles at a number of loci that interact either at the level of gene expression or via gene products.

Table 3: Principal Investigations Recommended in the Assessment of Pulmonary Hypertension

Pulmonary function tests

Full spirometry and CO diffusion studies are necessary to differentiate obstructive or restrictive pathology. Express data as % predicted, corrected for haematocrit. Reduction in transfer factor is the most sensitive test for pulmonary vascular disease, especially if disproportionately severe compared with reduced FVC. FEV1, FVC, TLC, Dlco, Kco should all be assessed.

Doppler echocardiography

Haemodynamic assessment
- Tricuspid regurgitation velocity (most accurate echocardiographic technique for estimating peak PAP
- Right ventricular outflow tract flow acceleration time
- Pulmonary artery systolic flow acceleration time
- Right ventricular ejection time
- Right ventricular index of myocardial performance
- Timing of mid systolic deceleration of right ventricular ejection
- Right ventricle long axis function (marker of overall right ventricular systolic function)

Qualitative assessment
- Enlarged right atrium and ventricle
- Right ventricular hypertrophy
- D shaped left ventricular cavity with interventricular septum flattening in systole
- Diminished atrial wave of the pulmonary valve
- Mid-systolic closure or notching of pulmonary valve

Right heart catheterisation
The following variables should be measured:
- Right atrial pressure
- Right ventricular systolic and end-diastolic pressure
- Pulmonary artery systolic, diastolic and mean pressure
- Pulmonary capillary wedge pressure
- Systemic and pulmonary arterial oxygen saturation
- Cardiac output

Vasodilator testing
- Recommended using intravenous iloprost/epoprostanol or adenosine or inhaled nitric oxide
Positive if > 10mm Hg fall in mean PAP and no change or increase in cardiac output.

In familial PAH this appears to involve mutations in a member of the TGFb superfamily of receptors[10,11] and a smaller number of cases where the association is with the AIK1 receptor an accessory of TGFb receptor[12,13]. Studies have not suggested that either of these loci are involved as susceptibility alleles for SSc-associated PAH[14] but it is recognised that altered expression of TGFb superfamily receptors, interacting proteins or downstream signalling molecules occur in scleroderma itself and therefore may have relevance to the associated PAH.

Other factors may play a part. There is evidence of widespread endothelial cell (EC) activation or damage in SSc and this may be the earliest lesion[14]. Markers of EC activation have been reported to be elevated in SSC-associate PAH suggesting the possibility that early EC pathology may be important[15,16].

End-stage PAH shows widespread medial and adventitial fibrosis, proliferative lesions and intimal hyperplasia and luminal obliteration: a highly complex pathology. Interestingly, the histology of digital arteries is very similar to that of PAH with medial and advential fibrosis leading to structural luminal narrowing[17].

There are also some histologigenic factors. Deficiency in natural vasodilators such as endothelium derived nitric oxide or excessive vasoconstrictors such as endothelin-1 might contribute to pathogenesis.

The vascular manifestations of SSc all have a vasospastic element but it does not seem that reversible vasospasm is the major process underlying established PAH lesions. Defects in the balance of vasoconstrictors and vasodilators may be important and it is notable that effective agents in the treatment of these complications (prostcyclin analogues, endothelin receptor blockers and ACEIs for SRC) all have vasodilatory properties.

Elevated levels of the potent vasoconstrictor ET-1 are a feature of SSc associated PAH[18]. It has been suggested that altered sensitivity of voltage gated potassium channels in the pulmonary arterial smooth muscle may be involved in initiation or progression of primary pulmonary arterial hypertension[19].

All SSc patients have Raynaud's phenomenon and so almost certainly exhibit defects in vasomotor regulation. It is possible that the less severely involved vessels may be vasodilated and that some of the short term benefits of therapy occur in this way. It is very unlikely to be a prominent longer term mechanism as the time-course of improvement is generally over days or weeks and some form of structural remodelling is much more likely.

It is interesting that endothelin receptor blockade is antifibrotic[20] and also that iloprost appears to downregulate expression of a potentially important downstream profibrotic mediator connective tissue growth factor (CTGF)[21].

Treatment of PAH

The development of treatments of proven efficacy for PAH is a major milestone for SSc management. Historically pulmonary hypertension therapies were confined to treatment with vasodilators including calcium channel blockers, which were rarely effective in scleroderma patients.

Oxygen was provided either intermittently for exertional dyspnoea or later in the disease as long term (16h per day) low flow oxygen aiming to reduce or reverse hypoxia induced pulmonary vasodilation[22]. Right heart failure was treated conventionally with care to avoid over-diuresis, but the long term outlook was dire and few scleroderma patients, on a global basis, received a transplanted lung or heart-lung.

The development of long-term parenteral prostacyclin analogue infusions, originally envisioned as a "bridge to transplantation," was found in a seminal prospective placebo controlled clinical trial to be an effective therapy. This trial involved patients with primary pulmonary hypertension who were treated for 16 weeks. The results were dramatic. There was improvement in exercise capacity with treatment but also significant mortality benefit even in this small study[23].

This landmark trial was later repeated for patients with connective tissue disease associated hypertension and again positive results were obtained although this time with trends but no statistically significant mortality benefit[24]. More recent studies have also shown benefit for the subcutaneous prostacyclin analogue treprostinil[25] and for nebulised agents given by inhalation[26]. The robust nature of these responses provides important proof of concept support for prostacyclin metabolism and signalling being important in the pathogenesis of PAH.

The orally active endothelin receptor blocker Bosentan has also been shown to be efficacious. This drug was originally developed for more common forms of cardiovascular disease but a recent prospective placebo controlled trial showed beneficial effects in both primary and connective tissue disease associated pulmonary arterial hypertension[27, 28].

In North America and Europe licensed therapies for PAH now include parenteral prostacyclin analogues (epoprostanol and iloprost, and remodulin) and oral bosentan. Other studies to refine and integrate these therapies are presently underway, including selective phosphodiesterase inhibitors such as sildenafil[29].

The major limitation to these treatments is cost. Other specific problems include line sepsis and the catastrophic effect of pump failure and acute withdrawal of prostanoids in established patients and the general problems of long-term ambulatory central venous catheterisation.

Current Management

Care pathways for patients with SSc related PAH are now being developed and one such pathway is shown in **Figure 1**. These care pathways are likely to be refined and modified but it is a tremendous advance upon the available approaches of just a few years ago. A major goal at present is education of the medical community, patients and their carer, and integration of care between pulmonologists, cardiologists and rheumatologists.

There are now established protocols and clinical support infrastructure to allow effective administration of advanced therapies for SSc associated PAH. Surgical options remain, notably atrial septostomy and transplantation for end-stage disease[30, 31].

Specialised centres in the UK now coordinate management from the stage of right heart catheterisation. If therapeutic benefit of earlier treatment is shown then decentralisation of care will be increasingly possible.

The major focus over the next few years should be definition of identification of early stage pulmonary vascular disease with prevention rather than treatment of Class III and IV disease.

References

1.   Coghlan JG, Mukerjee D. The heart and pulmonary vasculature in scleroderma: clinical features and pathobiology. Curr Opin Rheumatol. 2001 Nov;13(6):495-9. Review.

2.   Young RH, Mark GJ. Pulmonary vascular changes in scleroderma. Am J Med. 1978 Jun;64(6):998-1004.

3.   Sackner MA, Heinz ER, Steinberg AJ. The heart in scleroderma. Am J Cardiol. 1966.

4.   Mukerjee D, St George D, Coleiro B, Knight C, Denton CP, Davar J, Black CM, Coghlan JG. Prevalence and outcome in systemic sclerosis associated pulmonary arterial hypertension: application of a registry approach. Ann Rheum Dis. 2003, 62:1088-93.

Figure 1: Algorithm for Management of Pulmonary Arterial Hypertension. This algorithm is based upon the consensus guidelines recently established in the UK by cardiologists, rheumatologists and respiratory physicians.

Clinical suspicion
Breathlessness
Syncope
Chest pain

Diagnosis
Doppler-echocardiography
Chest X ray (CXR)
Echocardiogram (ECG)
Pulmonary function tests (PFT)
Right heart catheter (RHC)
(resting mean PAP > 25mm Hg
or exercise PAP > 30 mm Hg)

Routine screening
Annual assessment in
limited cutaneous SSc
patients

Differential diagnosis
Ascertain pulmonary fibrosis
Exclude thromboembolic disease
Determine pulmonary venous
hypertension[1]

Risk stratification
NYHA grading of symptoms**
Submaximal exercise test (e.g. six minute walk)
Vasodilator challenge #
    peak and mean PA pressure
    cardiac index
    pulmonary vascular resistance

Therapy

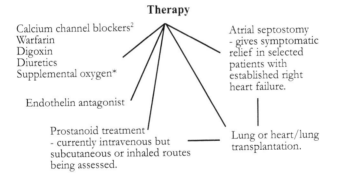

Calcium channel blockers[2]
Warfarin
Digoxin
Diuretics
Supplemental oxygen*

Endothelin antagonist

Prostanoid treatment
- currently intravenous but
subcutaneous or inhaled routes
being assessed.

Atrial septostomy
- gives symptomatic
relief in selected
patients with
established right
heart failure.

Lung or heart/lung
transplantation.

[1] definitively excluded by normal pulmonary capillary wedge pressure at right heart catheterization
[2] most patients with SSc are either intolerant due to gastroesophageal reflux or are already taking them
* long term oxygen therapy if average nocturnal arterial oxygen saturation falls below 90% on air
**New York Heart Association functional classification of pulmonary hypertension - Classes I asymptomatic to IV showing severe symptoms at rest with right heart failure
prostacyclin analogue, inhaled nitric oxide or intravenous adenosine may be used. Positive if 20% fall in PAP, PVR without fall in CO.

❖❖❖

5.   MacGregor AJ, Canavan R, Knight C, Denton CP, Davar J, Coghlan J, Black CM. Pulmonary hypertension in systemic sclerosis: risk factors for progression and consequences for survival. Rheumatology. 2001 Apr;40(4):453-9.

6.   Mukerjee D, St George D, Knight C, Davar J, Wells AU, Du Bois RM, Black CM, Coghlan JG. Echocardiography and pulmonary function as screening tests for pulmonary arterial hypertension in systemic sclerosis. Rheumatology (Oxford). 2004, 43(4):461-6.

7.   Denton CP, Cailes JB, Phillips GD, Wells AU, Black CM, Bois RM. Comparison of Doppler echocardiography and right heart catheterization to assess pulmonary hypertension in systemic sclerosis. Br J Rheumatol. 1997 Feb;36(2):239-43.

8.   Chemla D, Castelain V, Herve P, Lecarpentier Y, Brimioulle S. Haemodynamic evaluation of pulmonary hypertension. Eur Respir J. 2002 Nov;20(5):1314-31.

9.   British Cardiac Society Guidelines: Recommendations on the management of pulmonary hypertension in clinical practice.Heart. 2001 Sep;86 Suppl 1:I1-13.

10. Rudarakanchana N, Flanagan JA, Chen H, Upton PD, Machado R, Patel D, Trembath RC, Morrell NW. Functional analysis of bone morphogenetic protein type II receptor mutations underlying primary pulmonary hypertension. Hum Mol Genet. 2002 Jun 15;11(13):1517-25.

11. Trembath RC, Thomson JR, Machado RD, Morgan NV, Atkinson C, Winship I, Simonneau G, Galie N, Loyd JE, Humbert M, Nichols WC, Morrell NW, Berg J, Manes A, McGaughran J, Pauciulo M, Wheeler L. Clinical and molecular genetic features of pulmonary hypertension in patients with hereditary hemorrhagic telangiectasia. N Engl J Med. 2001 Aug 2;345(5):325-34.

12. Trembath RC. Mutations in the TGF-beta type 1 receptor, ALK1, in combined primary pulmonary hypertension and hereditary haemorrhagic telangiectasia, implies pathway specificity. J Heart Lung Transplant. 2001 Feb;20(2):175.

13. Morse J, Barst R, Horn E, Cuervo N, Deng Z, Knowles J. Pulmonary hypertension in scleroderma spectrum of disease: lack of bone morphogenetic protein receptor 2 mutations. J Rheumatol. 2002 Nov;29(11):2379-81.

14. Crilly A, Hamilton J, Clark CJ, Jardine A, Madhok R. Analysis of transforming growth factor beta1 gene polymorphisms in patients with systemic sclerosis. Ann Rheum Dis. 2002 Aug;61(8):678-81.

15. Stratton RJ, Pompon L, Coghlan JG, Pearson JD, Black CM. Soluble thrombomodulin concentration is raised in scleroderma associated pulmonary hypertension. Ann Rheum Dis. 2000 Feb;59(2):132-4.

16. Stratton RJ, Coghlan JG, Pearson JD, Burns A, Sweny P, Abraham DJ, Black CM. Different patterns of endothelial cell activation in renal and pulmonary vascular disease in scleroderma. QJM. 1998 Aug;91(8):561-6.

17. Yi ES, Kim H, Ahn H, Strother J, Morris T, Masliah E, Hansen LA, Park K, Friedman PJ. Distribution of obstructive intimal lesions and their cellular phenotypes in chronic pulmonary hypertension. A morphometric and immunohistochemical study. Am J Respir Crit Care Med. 2000 Oct;162(4 Pt 1):1577-86.

18. Vancheeswaran R, Magoulas T, Efrat G, Wheeler-Jones C, Olsen I, Penny R, Black CM. Circulating endothelin-1 levels in systemic sclerosis subsets—a marker of fibrosis or vascular dysfunction? J Rheumatol. 1994 Oct;21(10):1838-44.

19. Yuan JX, Aldinger AM, Juhaszova M, Wang J, Conte JV Jr, Gaine SP, Orens JB, Rubin LJ. Dysfunctional voltage-gated K+ channels in pulmonary artery smooth muscle cells of patients with primary pulmonary hypertension. Circulation. 1998 Oct 6;98(14):1400-6.

20. Shi-Wen X, Denton CP, Dashwood MR, Holmes AM, Bou-Gharios G, Pearson JD, Black CM, Abraham DJ. Fibroblast matrix gene expression and connective tissue remodeling: role of endothelin-1. J Invest Dermatol. 2001 Mar;116(3):417-25.

21. Stratton R, Shiwen X, Martini G, Holmes A, Leask A, Haberberger T, Martin GR, Black CM, Abraham D. Iloprost suppresses connective tissue growth factor production in fibroblasts and in the skin of scleroderma patients. J Clin Invest. 2001 Jul;108(2):241-50.

22. Roberts DH, Lepore JJ, Maroo A, Semigran MJ, Ginns LC. Oxygen therapy improves cardiac index and pulmonary vascular resistance in patients with pulmonary hypertension. Chest. 2001 Nov;120(5):1547-55.

23. Barst RJ, Rubin LJ, Long WA, McGoon MD, Rich S, Badesch DB, Groves BM, Tapson VF, Bourge RC, Brundage BH, et al. A comparison of continuous intravenous epoprostenol (prostacyclin) with conventional therapy for primary pulmonary hypertension. The Primary Pulmonary Hypertension Study Group. N Engl J Med. 1996 Feb 1;334(5):296-302.

24. Badesch DB, Tapson VF, McGoon MD, Brundage BH, Rubin LJ, Wigley FM, Rich S, Barst RJ, Barrett PS, Kral KM, Jobsis MM, Loyd JE, Murali S, Frost A, Girgis R, Bourge RC, Ralph DD, Elliott CG, Hill NS, Langleben D, Schilz RJ, McLaughlin VV, Robbins IM, Groves BM, Shapiro S, Medsger TA Jr. Continuous intravenous epoprostenol for pulmonary hypertension due to the scleroderma spectrum of disease. A randomized, controlled trial. Ann Intern Med. 2000 Mar 21;132(6):425-34.

25. Simonneau G, Barst RJ, Galie N, Naeije R, Rich S, Bourge RC, Keogh A, Oudiz R, Frost A, Blackburn SD, Crow JW, Rubin LJ. Continuous subcutaneous infusion of treprostinil, a prostacyclin analogue, in patients with pulmonary arterial hypertension: a double-blind, randomized, placebo-controlled trial. Am J Respir Crit Care Med. 2002 Mar 15;165(6):800-4.

26. Olschewski H, Simonneau G, Galie N, Higenbottam T, Naeije R, Rubin LJ, Nikkho S, Speich R, Hoeper MM, Behr J, Winkler J, Sitbon O, Popov W, Ghofrani HA, Manes A, Kiely DG, Ewert R, Meyer A, Corris PA, Delcroix M, Gomez-Sanchez M, Siedentop H, Seeger W. Inhaled iloprost for severe pulmonary hypertension. N Engl J Med. 2002 Aug 1;347(5):322-9.

27. Channick RN, Simonneau G, Sitbon O, Robbins IM, Frost A, Tapson VF, Badesch DB, Roux S, Rainisio M, Bodin F, Rubin LJ. Effects of the dual endothelin-receptor antagonist bosentan in patients with pulmonary hypertension: a randomised placebo-controlled study. Lancet. 2001 Oct 6;358(9288):1119-23.

28. Rubin LJ, Badesch DB, Barst RJ, Galie N, Black CM, Keogh A, Pulido T, Frost A, Roux S, Leconte I, Landzberg M, Simonneau G. Bosentan therapy for pulmonary arterial hypertension. N Engl J Med. 2002 Mar 21;346(12):896-903.

29. Ghofrani HA, Wiedemann R, Rose F, Schermuly RT, Olschewski H, Weissmann N, Gunther A, Walmrath D, Seeger W, Grimminger F. Sildenafil for treatment of lung fibrosis and pulmonary hypertension: a randomised controlled trial. Lancet. 2002 Sep 21;360(9337):895-900.

30. Allcock RJ, O'Sullivan JJ, Corris PA. Palliation of systemic sclerosis-associated pulmonary hypertension by atrial septostomy. Arthritis Rheum. 2001 Jul;44(7): 1660-2.

31. Rosas V, Conte JV, Yang SC, Gaine SP, Borja M, Wigley FM, White B, Orens JB. Lung transplantation and systemic sclerosis. Ann Transplant. 2000;5(3):38-43. Review.

Molière, Maurice Raynaud
and Modern Measures of the Microcirculation
by Kevin J. Howell

Kevin Howell is a Clinical Scientist for Professor Black at the Royal Free Hospital in London. He began working in the field of scleroderma in 1991, and uses the techniques of capillaroscopy and infrared thermography.

"That must be wonderful: I don't understand it at all!"

When the Parisian playwright Molière (1622-1675) wrote these words, he presumably wasn't referring to the human blood circulation. Yet to those of us who are studying the function of the very smallest blood vessels in the twenty-first century, the quotation can seem at times rather appropriate.

Our microscopic blood vessels, which make up the *microcirculation*, are critically important. They deliver blood rich in oxygen on the final part of its journey to the organs of the body, including the skin. They are also a delivery system for a bewildering array of chemical substances secreted by the body into the bloodstream to regulate the control of those target organs.

Some of the vessels of the microcirculation can be influenced themselves by substances in the bloodstream. In response to these chemicals, a blood vessel might widen or narrow. Or a rather less obvious property of the vessel might change, such as its porosity or "leakiness." And we mustn't forget that some blood vessels are influenced not just by circulating chemicals, but by the nervous system too.

This intricate network of competing influences on small blood vessels helps the body cope with the rather daunting demands of daily life. The regulation of blood flow helps us to keep a similar blood pressure regardless of whether we are lying down or standing up, or to maintain a constant core body temperature at the expense of a very variable skin temperature.

The problem is, when one or more of these influences on the microcirculation starts to go wrong, it can be almost impossible to identify the smoking gun, given the complexity of the way our blood vessels work. Everyone agrees this complexity is truly wonderful. But in many respects, we don't really understand it at all! Yet.

It's unlikely that Molière would have been very sympathetic to the plight of modern-day doctors and researchers who are struggling to comprehend the microcirculation. He was a fierce critic of the medical profession, publishing a string of satirical plays in which the humour was at the expense of the Parisian well-to-do, and the physicians who sought, ineffectively, to treat their ailments. It is not surprising, though, that seventeenth century medicine was such a hit and miss affair given the very limited knowledge at the time about what was actually going on inside a patient's body.

Nowadays, we take all sorts of medical investigative procedures almost for granted, but in Molière's day, a physician had little information about his patient other than that which could be ascertained from an external examination and the symptoms of the condition.

Elsewhere in Europe during Molière's lifetime, Galileo (1564-1642) and then Newton (1643-1727) were putting forward ideas that would give birth to the science of physics. It was to take centuries before this new thinking about the nature of matter and energy gave rise to technology that could be applied to gain information about the anatomy and physiology of living patients.

For Molière, the wait for an X ray would have been around two hundred and fifty years; for an MRI scan it would have been in excess of three hundred years. With the benefit of hindsight, perhaps it was a little harsh of the playwright to be so scathing about doctors, given that they were working largely in ignorance of the internal workings of live subjects.

New beginnings: Raynaud takes an interest

In 1863 another Frenchman, Maurice Raynaud, published a book entitled *Doctors of the Time of Molière*. Raynaud was a physician with a particular interest in the history of medicine, and went on to get a further doctorate in letters for his historical research.

Raynaud could have called his book *Doctors in the seventeenth century*, but by invoking Molière he perhaps meant to make a point: that the most famous French critic of doctors hadn't really given the profession a fair or accurate hearing.

Doctors of the Time of Molière was a well-respected text. Charles Kingsley, author of *The Water Babies* and Professor of History at Cambridge, was a fan, but the book is now long forgotten.

We remember Raynaud for another reason. Just a year before his book was published, Raynaud had received his first doctorate in medicine for his thesis *Local Asphyxia and Symmetrical Gangrene of the Extremities*. Raynaud's description of colour change in fingers on exposure to cold was the first decent scientific appraisal of the phenomenon that now bears his name.

Raynaud's description of this "vasospasm" as we might nowadays call it cannot be faulted, but it was far more difficult to find an explanation for the condition. Raynaud studied the arteries of the fingers of some patients *post mortem*, and temporarily blocked the function of nerves in the spines of other patients to see what would happen.

But for the most part, Raynaud found himself no better off than a doctor of the time of Molière, two hundred years before. There was still no effective way to *measure* what was happening to patients.

Modern measurement—beginning to make sense of it all

The reality is that progress on the understanding of microcirculatory disorders like Raynaud's phenomenon has been slow to develop in the one hundred and forty years since Raynaud's thesis. But now, at last, things are beginning to change.

In this article I want to discuss the advances in technology of the last thirty years or so, that have revolutionised our ability to measure how the small blood vessels of the body are performing. Although there are now many ways of measuring the microcirculation, I will focus on just a few specific techniques.

This is not because I think the others are less useful or somehow inferior: the methods I will describe simply happen to be those that we have adopted here at the Royal Free Hospital. We believe these methods are a good way forward for learning about small blood vessels.

Imaging with heat

When I began working as a Clinical Scientist for Professor Black at the Royal Free Hospital in 1992, our centre already had some experience with *thermography*. My task was to develop thermography into an established and accepted method for assessing Raynaud's phenomenon routinely in our hospital. It was also quite clear that thermography would prove to be useful for the assessment of other rheumatological conditions.

Thermography, as the name implies, is simply imaging from heat. We all learned at school that heat moves around in three ways. Firstly, there is *conduction* through a material. This means to say that if I place a length of copper piping in a fire and hold onto the opposite end, it won't be long before I burn my hand!

Secondly, heat moves via the *convection* of fluids. Switch on a heater downstairs, and warm air will flow upstairs to heat the other rooms of the house a little. None of this, though, explains why sunlight feels warm on our faces, or a campfire can warm our hands.

We owe an explanation of heat transfer by *radiation* to William Herschel (1738-1822). Herschel is one of those great characters from history who defies categorisation. He was not just a fabled astronomer, but also a brilliant musician and, most relevant to our story, a highly competent experimental physicist.

In 1800, Herschel performed an experiment to study the heating effect on the eye of stars of different colours when observed through a telescope. He began by splitting sunlight into its constituent colours with a prism, and placing thermometers within the different coloured areas of the spectrum. This showed that the red end of the spectrum caused the greatest temperature rise.

But Herschel also found that a thermometer placed outside the visible part of the spectrum showed the highest temperatures of all. He called this phenomenon "dark heat," but nowadays we know this energy conveyed by radiation at frequencies beyond the visible red part of the spectrum as *infrared*.

William's son, John Herschel (1792-1871), took his father's work still further in 1840. He soaked a strip of paper in alcohol and coated it with lampblack, then placed the strip in sunlight for the whole day. The result was a rudimentary image varying from light to dark and progressing along the paper as the sun moved across the sky, obscured intermittently by clouds. This picture, drawn using heat, could be considered the first true *thermogram*.

Then, in the early part of the twentieth century, quantum mechanics gave us predictions about how infrared radiation should behave. These predictions were shown by experimenters to be extremely accurate: the nature of radiant heat was now understood. From now on, knowing the frequency of the radiation being detected and a few physical properties of the target, it would be possible to calculate the target's temperature.

The Second World War saw some early attempts to use infrared for military purposes. Since heat should still be detectable in, for example, dark or misty conditions, it might be a way to "see" when normally this was not possible. Early attempts at infrared detection as a navigation aid were soon abandoned, though. And true "imaging" of targets using infrared was not achieved until much later.

The Cold War saw a bigger effort on the infrared imaging front, and by the early 1950s, some basic "night-sight" technology was available to the military. As this became more refined and practicable in the 1960s, word of the technology began to reach the medical profession. Physicians have recognised the importance of temperature measurement since the dawn of medicine. It is known the ancient Egyptians associated fever with disease, and there is also an explicit reference to fever and disease in the book of Deuteronomy (28:22).

Carl Wunderlich (1815-1877) performed hundreds of temperature measurements on patients published in 1868. This work demonstrated that careful *measurement* of temperature gave physicians important information about a patient's state of health.

The advances in thermal imaging in the 1960s set many in the medical profession thinking. Now it was possible to measure temperature across the entire surface of the human skin, and represent this temperature distribution as an image. Better still, the technique involved no physical contact with the patient, and it was painless.

Would localised changes in skin surface temperature prove to be as useful as Wunderlich's measurements with simple thermometers? The science of *medical thermography* was born!

Modern thermal imagers are typically little bigger than a standard video camera, and almost as easy to use. The military demand for a compact and rugged device that could "see in the dark" has given us, after forty years of refinement, a product that is nearly perfect for medical use too. This is a good example of what some like to call *technology transfer:* developing an idea for one use, often military, but then applying it equally effectively for another.

Nowadays we can record a thermal image instantly, and the image can be stored and displayed on a standard office computer. Software allows us to work on the images and give them a colour coding so that, for example, the cooler areas in an image might be blue, and the warmer areas orange or red. We can also trace around any part of the image using the computer mouse, and the software will tell us the temperature in the area we have defined.

Some of the earliest work in medical thermography showed that breast tumours caused a raised skin temperature. Thermography also proved to be useful for looking at skin overlying inflamed joints in arthritic conditions. But it wasn't long before the technique was also applied to the study of

Raynaud's phenomenon, which, after all, is a condition where the skin temperature is clearly abnormal at times.

The most severe symptoms of Raynaud's phenomenon occur after exposure to cold, so in an attempt to maximise the difference between Raynaud's phenomenon patients and normal subjects, we perform a *cold challenge test* with thermography at the Royal Free Hospital. The test is proven to be helpful in the diagnosis and assessment of Raynaud's phenomenon. Professor Ring at the University of Glamorgan has, for example, around thirty years of experience in using a version of the cold challenge test, and has published his results widely.

The essence of the cold challenge test is that it measures a patient's response to a *change* in temperature of the hands. It may not be enough to simply measure the temperature of the hands when they are warm, and this is often the state the hands are in once the patient has been inside a nice warm hospital for an hour or two!

Physicians rarely see an attack of Raynaud's phenomenon in a clinic room. So if we are not to miss the point about Raynaud's phenomenon, we need to record infrared images from a patient not just when she has warm hands (I say "she" because more than eighty percent of our patients are female), but also after we have deliberately made her hands cold.

The patient is asked to rest in our laboratory for fifteen minutes, in order that she adapts to the room temperature which is always 23°C. Next we record an infrared image of both hands, to establish a *baseline* reading. Then the patient puts on a pair of light plastic gloves to keep the skin dry and places her hands in a bucket of water at 15°C for one minute. That's cold, but it's not unbearable! I should stress that the cold water rarely provokes a true attack of Raynaud's phenomenon with visible colour changes, but there is enough temperature change of the hands for the infrared camera to detect a difference.

With the hands removed from the water and the gloves, we then begin to record a sequence of infrared images of the hands over the following ten minutes. This establishes the *re-warming rate* of the hands.

So what do we find? Not surprisingly, Raynaud's phenomenon patients recover the temperature of their hands much more slowly than most healthy subjects.

A normal recovery time is within ten minutes, whereas the great majority of our patients are little warmer at the end of the ten-minute period than they were at the moment their hands left the cold water. In Raynaud's phenomenon, many of the smaller blood vessels in the skin of the fingers have a tendency to narrow more dramatically in the cold than normal. With very little warm blood flowing through these constricted vessels, there will be little or no re-warming of the hand.

While this sounds like something the patient might be able to describe to us unaided, we do believe it is very important to *document* this poor re-warming using thermography. A small number of our patients prove to have a good re-warming rate, and in some of these cases we might need to look for an alternative reason to explain their symptoms.

We are also beginning to learn about how to make use of some of the more subtle information the cold challenge test conveys. Raynaud's phenomenon is normally *bilateral*, by which I mean it affects both hands more or less equally.

Thermography easily shows us where this is not the case, and again we might need to consider an alternative diagnosis in some patients. Peripheral nerve entrapments, occurring perhaps at the wrist or elbow, will often affect the speed at which certain fingers of the hand re-warm.

As I mentioned at the beginning of my article, peripheral blood flow is in part controlled by the nervous system. The use of thermography to detect trapped nerves, especially in patients who might be unfortunate enough to suffer from Raynaud's phenomenon too, is an application that interests me very much. There is a little research already published on this question, but as a community of thermographers we have most of the work still to do on that one!

Some researchers have suggested that the cold challenge test can differentiate between patients with "primary" Raynaud's phenomenon, and those with Raynaud's phenomenon "secondary" to diseases such as scleroderma. It is certainly very difficult to draw such an inference from the study of an individual patient. But if there are differences, on average, in the way large groups of primary and secondary Raynaud's patients re-warm, then that might help us understand how or even if the two types of Raynaud's phenomenon are different.

One evident weakness of the cold challenge test is its tendency to show that some completely healthy subjects, who do not complain of Raynaud's phenomenon, are very slow to re-warm their hands. In other words, we get some *false-positive* results.

I think this teaches us to be conservative in interpreting what the cold challenge test really tells us. Cold challenge will highlight quite reliably which of our patients suffer from *vasospasm*, that troublesome tendency towards overly constricted small blood vessels in the cold. And without vasospasm, a patient will not suffer attacks of Raynaud's phenomenon. But many people will suffer from vasospasm without ever really developing the true symptoms of Raynaud's phenomenon. They seem to be spared the colour changes and numb fingers, although their hands are very cold. Thermography, of course, cannot differentiate between this group of people, and true Raynaud's phenomenon sufferers.

This raises the question of what Raynaud's phenomenon really is! While we would all like to think that a patient either has a particular condition or not, is healthy or unwell, in the case of Raynaud's phenomenon the diagnosis depends on how we ask the question.

There are no hard and fast rules defined for diagnosing Raynaud's phenomenon, and factors like the frequency of attacks and the colour changes observed vary enormously from patient to patient. Whilst some hospital patients clearly have severe Raynaud's phenomenon, and others might be entirely free of symptoms, a great number reside in a grey area of mild intolerance to the cold and infrequent colour change. It is in this grey area that perhaps the cold challenge test can be of most use, to demonstrate that the underlying vasospasm is either mild, or perhaps more significant.

The doctor involved in the diagnosis of Raynaud's phenomenon will always need to make that diagnosis primarily on the basis of the symptoms of the patient. But cold challenge is the most effective and convenient physiological test we have to support a diagnosis of Raynaud's phenomenon.

We have also started to use thermography at the Royal Free Hospital for the assessment of *localised scleroderma*, which is sometimes called *morphoea*. As its name suggests, localised scleroderma just involves hardening of the skin in patches or *plaques*, rather than the more widespread skin changes and internal organ involvement seen in systemic scleroderma.

Localised scleroderma begins more commonly in children than in adults, and there is the risk that limbs may become deformed around these areas of hard skin, which do not extend as the child grows.

In 1992, Nina Birdi and her colleagues in Toronto published work which indicated that thermography is very effective for assessing morphoea plaques. They showed that plaques that are still extending, and therefore require treatment, show up as hot on an infrared image.

In other words, there is more blood flowing in these areas than in normal skin: active morphoea skin is *inflamed*. Birdi also showed that morphoea that has ceased to extend is no longer any hotter than normal skin: the inflammation has gone away.

In October 2002 my colleague Giorgia Martini, now back in Padua after her stay in London at the Royal Free and Great Ormond Street hospitals, published our own findings on thermography as a tool for assessing morphoea. We agree that thermography is an excellent imaging technique for morphoea.

We use it regularly nowadays to provide supporting evidence of whether a morphoea plaque is likely to be active or not. If it is, the doctors might want to give an anti-inflammatory to combat the disease. Thermography can also show us, over a period of months, how well treatments are doing in reducing the temperature in these plaques. We take careful consideration of our infrared images before deciding that a plaque is inactive and stopping medication.

It is quite easy to make sense of an infrared image: the areas that are hotter than they should be are obvious on inspection. And if two trained observers are independently shown a selection of infrared images of morphoea plaques, they come to remarkably similar conclusions about which plaques look hot, and which are cold. This is an important finding because it tells us the technique may be reproduced by different people.

But it's not all good news. We have evidence that thermography also has limitations. While morphoea thickens the skin near the surface, in some cases it also seems to cause a *thinning* of the tissue deeper in the skin. For example, some patients have a reduced thickness of the fat layer at the base of the skin. Since this layer of fat is a rather good insulating material, it would be naïve of us to imagine that there is no effect on skin surface temperature if the layer thins. There is better conduction of the heat from deep within the human body to the skin surface in places where this fat layer is thin or missing.

The upshot of this is that plaques of morphoea overlying areas with thinning of the fat layer are hot in an infrared image. But the plaque may not be *inflamed* at all: this is simply heat that has found its way to the skin surface more easily than we would normally expect. However, it is not easy to tell where this thinning of the fat layer is occurring, so we cannot always know whether to believe the plaque really has increased blood flow, or is just hot because of conduction from deeper tissues.

This is a fundamental weakness of thermography: it measures skin *temperature*, whereas what we are really interested in is skin *blood flow*. Although there are lots of situations where the two quantities reflect each other, our experience with morphoea reminds us this is not always true.

Ideally, we need an imaging technique that has all the speed, ease-of-use and cost benefits of thermography, but gives us a direct measure of *blood flow*.

Does such a technique exist? Well, our friends in industry are certainly working towards it!

Towards a convenient, true measure of blood flow in skin

In 1975, a theoretical physicist by the name of Michael Stern at the National Heart and Lung Institute in the US was looking into ways of using laser light to measure the blood flowing in the microcirculation.

One property of laser light is that of *coherence*, which is a way of saying that the light in a laser beam is perfectly lined-up or in step. This coherent light stays in a narrow beam, and it is also a very pure colour or *frequency*.

Stern placed an elastic band tightly around the base of his finger to impede the circulation, and illuminated the fingertip with a laser. The light passing through the finger, and projecting onto a piece of card behind, twinkled in a *speckle pattern*, which Stern expected to see when coherent light travelled through a complicated stationary structure like a finger.

Next he removed the elastic band, and blood flowed back into the finger. Light still went right through the finger to reach the cardboard, but now the speckle pattern was gone! What had happened to turn pure, coherent laser light into everyday, jumbled-up light incapable of producing a speckle pattern?

Stern recognised that the answer lay in the fact that blood, or more precisely the red cells within it, are moving and acting as scatterers of the laser light. And any scatterer that is *moving* will change the *frequency* of the light, and hence its colour.

Christian Doppler (1803-1853) first described this effect in 1842, and at school we are all taught a little bit about the *Doppler effect*. This change in frequency due to movement is why a police car siren has a different pitch when it is moving towards us to when it is moving away.

Similarly, astronomers have observed a distinct reddening of faraway galaxies—evidence that the distant universe is receding from us at fantastic speed. But the effect on the colour of light caused by a *Doppler shift* cannot be seen if an object is moving at everyday speeds.

In fact, by the time of Stern's experiment, researchers had been using tiny Doppler shifts of laser light to measure the flow of blood in large blood vessels for more than ten years. But measuring the blood flow in a large vessel was a different and simpler problem compared to Stern's challenge. A large vessel like an artery is wide enough to encompass the entire width of the laser beam, so we can be sure our measurements come only from the flow in that single vessel.

But Stern's set-up is not like illuminating a single artery at all. His laser beam is illuminating many tiny blood vessels within the skin all at once.

Some of these vessels will be slightly wider than others, and they will all be oriented differently to each other in the skin. The upshot of this is that Stern's laser-Doppler experiment gives not just one Doppler shift of the laser light, representing one rate of flow of the blood, but a huge number of Doppler shifts. This is indicative of red blood cells circulating around inside the skin in a wide variety of directions at many different speeds.

Put another way, there is a *spectrum* of Doppler shifts arising from the flow of blood in the microcirculation.

Stern and his colleagues set out to build equipment that would measure this Doppler spectrum, and interpret it to give a result that indicated the average blood flow within the illuminated skin. This is the basis of the *laser Doppler flowmeters* that are on the market today.

A modern laser Doppler flowmeter consists of a small, portable box of electronics where the laser is housed, and a length of fibre-optic to carry the laser light to the patient. A small probe at the end of the fibre-optic sticks to the patient's skin.

It is this probe that both illuminates a small area of skin with laser light, and collects some of the Doppler-shifted light, which is reflected from the skin and sent back down the fibre optic to the processing electronics. A small display on the base unit gives a live readout of the amount of blood flowing in the skin. All the information can be piped to an attached computer, from which we can graph the data and print out results.

Laser Doppler flowmetry, often called just *LDF* is now well established in microvascular research, and that very much includes the study of

Raynaud's phenomenon and scleroderma. At the Royal Free Hospital we have used LDF to look at blood flow in the fingers of Raynaud's phenomenon patients after our old friend, the cold water challenge to the hands.

It is perhaps not surprising that we find our patients have lower blood flow and a delayed recovery compared to healthy subjects, but some of the detail in our results is a bit less obvious.

For example, it seems that the *speed* of red blood cells is rather similar in the skin of Raynaud's phenomenon patients and healthy people, but the *concentration* of red cells is quite different. Only LDF can give us information as detailed as that instantaneously.

Elsewhere in the UK, there is great interest in LDF at university teaching hospitals in Dundee, Manchester and Bath. Studies performed on Raynaud's phenomenon have included looking at blood flow in response to skin heating, skin cooling and applying drugs to the skin surface that ought to widen the blood vessels in the skin beneath.

Some drugs that aren't normally well absorbed by the skin can be coaxed through by applying a very small electric current across the skin. This shows the versatility of LDF as a research tool in experienced hands.

I have discussed the blood flow in skin so far, but special fibre optics available for laser Doppler flow meters can be introduced almost anywhere in the body, so that we can attempt to measure blood flow in internal organs. This facility is very useful in scleroderma research.

There has long been debate about what is happening to the internal organs in scleroderma. Everyone agrees that some organs suffer a degree of *fibrosis* very much like the thickening of skin that is evident in patients externally. But is there a reduction in blood flow in internal organs too, much like the Raynaud's phenomenon that happens in the skin of the fingers? Are some of the symptoms patients suffer internally due to lack of blood flow?

The jury is still out on these questions, but we have certainly begun to look for some answers. I spent a short period some years ago using LDF to measure blood flow in the bowels of some scleroderma patients.

We were able to introduce the fibre-optic into the bowel along a flexible endoscope while the patient had a routine endoscopy performed. Of course, we did not find this an easy technique to perform, and the results are difficult to make sense of. But there was certainly no conclusive evidence that scleroderma patients lack blood flow in the bowel, and my money is on bowel symptoms being due primarily to other effects, like fibrosis and an over-rich population of bacteria in the bowel.

The very latest laser-Doppler innovations are taking our knowledge of the microcirculation to a new level. For a few years now, so called *laser Doppler imagers* have been on the market.

These systems move a single laser beam across an areaof skin, up and down, and left-to-right. From each point in the scan area, the Doppler information is reflected back to the instrument, and the blood flow is calculated for that position.

We can produce almost seven thousand of Michael Stern's single blood flow measurements, taken from across an area of skin. Each blood flow reading is turned into a point on an image, coloured according to its value.

Here, then is the first true *image* of blood flow in the small vessels of the skin—a very exciting development. Laser Doppler flow images can show us the blood flow across the entire hand in Raynaud's phenomenon studies.

This may also be a helpful technique in the study of morphoea—a way to clarify if those troublesome skin plaques with missing fat underneath really *are* hot due to increased blood flow, or simply because heat has reached the skin surface more easily in less insulated areas. This is the kind of work that will occupy me, and others with similar interests around the world, in the next few years.

The way ahead

When Lincoln Steffens returned from Russia in 1919, he commented, "I have seen the future, and it works!" but Russian Communism has not endured. We should be very wary of commenting on the future, because it hasn't happened yet!

Both patients and health professionals get frustrated at times at how complicated diseases like Raynaud's phenomenon and scleroderma appear to be. It seems modern medicine has defeated many of the easy diseases, but there are a bunch of conditions which are a lot harder to crack, and these remain rather mysterious.

It is impossible to know how quickly the medical profession will develop a full understanding of the microcirculation, and the things that go wrong with small blood vessels. But what I have described in this article, the progress in *physiological measurement* of the microcirculation in recent years, is just one of the many things in this book which I hope gives the reader reason to be optimistic. There can be no guarantees about the rate of our progress in future, but it is wonderful to contemplate that our knowledge about small blood vessels, and how to investigate them, is growing at a faster rate right now than at any time in history.

Having chastised soothsayers I will, nonetheless, make a few very conservative predictions about the future of microvascular research. Firstly, the big progress in Raynaud's phenomenon and scleroderma treatment will not come from clinical scientists like me, but instead from more "pure" researchers who are experts in subjects like immunology, pharmacology and genetics. But it will be down to people like me to prove that their ideas really do improve the lot of patients, to *measure* the influence future treatments have.

Secondly, our ability to measure is bound to improve, and it will be technology driven. In twenty years we will use technology that hasn't yet been invented to probe the physiology of patients.

Thirdly, all of this technology will be, just as it is now, expensive. This is a problem not unique to my field, but one destined to trouble the entire healthcare system worldwide. It is something our political leaders, particularly those with their hands on the purse strings, will need to address with increasing urgency in the next few years.

Lastly, the great credit for progress in Raynaud's and scleroderma research will justifiably go to the patients themselves. Our patients are, in my experience, extremely well informed about the importance of research. They recognise the need for studies involving themselves to further our knowledge, and I am always amazed at their continued willingness to actively participate in trials. Everybody also appreciates that it is patients who raise a significant proportion of the money that goes to fund research.

I hope this article has given just a flavour of my work as a Clinical Scientist on the microcirculation. It is certainly very stimulating work, and I rarely experience a day in which I find more answers than new questions! But that is a pretty good definition of rewarding work for a scientist, I feel!

◆ ❖ ◆

Introduction to Scleroderma Fibroblasts
by Maria Trojanowska, Ph.D.

Dr. Maria Trojanowska is Associate Professor, Division of Rheumatology and Immunology at the Medical University of South Carolina. The main area of research in her laboratory is regulation of extracellular matrix (ECM) deposition in healthy tissues and its dysregulation in diseases.

What did we learn by studying scleroderma fibroblasts?

In 2002, the scleroderma research community lost one of its most prominent members, Dr. E. Carwile LeRoy. Dr. LeRoy was one of the pioneers in scleroderma research, and was well known and admired around the world. He devoted his entire career to unraveling this complex disease. I was privileged to work with Carwile for a number of years and would like to dedicate this article to his memory.

Scleroderma fibroblast takes center stage

In 1972, LeRoy published his seminal observation that fibroblasts isolated from the skin of scleroderma patients produce more collagen than fibroblasts isolated from the skin of healthy people. The spindle-shaped fibroblasts are the specialized cells in the skin and other organs responsible for making connective tissue (also called extra cellular matrix).

Collagen, the most abundant protein in the human body, is a main component of the connective tissue. Although it was known that more collagen was deposited in the skin of scleroderma patients, giving the skin its characteristic tight and hidebound appearance, LeRoy's discovery had several important implications.

First, it suggested that abnormally activated fibroblasts residing in the skin of scleroderma patients are the culprits responsible for the augmented deposition of collagen in the skin.

Second, because scleroderma fibroblasts remained activated outside the living skin during culturing in the laboratory, it suggested that this defect is an intrinsic property of scleroderma fibroblasts. It was now possible to study this defect in the laboratory and to ask what causes the activated state of scleroderma cells.

Finally and most importantly, this finding generated hope that once we fully understand the specific defect of scleroderma fibroblast, treatments can be devised to revert the behavior of scleroderma fibroblasts back to normal. Indeed, LeRoy's publication has inspired a number of researchers around the world, including our laboratory in Charleston, South Carolina to pursue these questions.

I would also point out that the research on scleroderma fibroblasts has contributed significantly to other disease research in general, including many forms of fibrotic disease and cancer. Conversely, scleroderma researchers have always been in the forefront to apply any new knowledge and scientific tools to the study of scleroderma. Although we do not yet have all the answers, tremendous progress has been made in understanding the activation of scleroderma fibroblasts. In the next few sections I will describe our current understanding of scleroderma and discuss the challenges that still remain.

Scleroderma fibroblasts are indeed very different from healthy skin fibroblasts

In the years that followed LeRoy's discovery, many other proteins, besides collagen were found to be produced at abnormal levels by scleroderma fibroblasts, when compared to healthy fibroblasts.

Scleroderma fibroblasts overproduced most, if not all, of the components of the connective tissue. Other proteins including growth factors, cell surface receptors, signaling molecules and transcription factors were also synthesized at higher levels. Thus, scleroderma fibroblasts were indeed very different from healthy skin fibroblasts.

Because of technological advances we may soon know all of the proteins that are inappropriately produced by scleroderma fibroblasts. The recent sequencing of the human genome has given rise to new and exciting technologies, including DNA microarrays, which revolutionized the way in which gene expression is analyzed. This new technology allows for the simultaneous comparison of thousands of mRNAs (which are the blueprints for making proteins) from different samples.

Several scleroderma investigators are currently applying this new technology to catalogue all the differently produced mRNAs between scleroderma and healthy skin fibroblasts. Although their findings are preliminary, these studies suggest that several hundred mRNAs may be differently expressed by scleroderma fibroblasts.

Such studies are very labor intensive and verification of all of these mRNAs will take additional time. However, once this task is finished we will gain invaluable insight into the differences between scleroderma and healthy fibroblasts, thus bringing to fruition LeRoy's initial discovery made over thirty years ago.

One may ask why this knowledge is important and how can it help scleroderma patients? These comprehensive analyses may give physicians additional tools to diagnose patients with scleroderma and hopefully make a better prediction for the course of a disease. This, in turn, may help to design the best treatment for a particular group of patients.

Similar types of comprehensive analyses have recently been applied to patients with breast cancer. In this case, DNA microarray analyses helped to identify a group of genes referred to as "signatures" that characterize tumors with the potential to metastasize to other organs. Most importantly, these signature genes can be detected even in small primary tumors.

This method was a much more powerful predictor of disease outcome than any other standard method. This new tool will help physicians to identify very early the patients with poor prognosis and treat these patients more aggressively.

What causes scleroderma fibroblasts to make more collagen?

The behavior of scleroderma fibroblasts characterized by an excessive production of extracellular matrix proteins suggested that these cells are permanently "turned on."

Another area of intense research pursued by many investigators in the scleroderma field is to uncover what causes scleroderma fibroblasts to "turn on" and become high collagen producing cells. Clues to this mystery have come from advances in understanding how cells regulate protein synthesis.

Cellular protein synthesis is very tightly regulated at many levels to ensure proper cell function. The first regulatory step takes place in the cell nucleus. Here, the master blueprints for all proteins, called genes, are stored in the form of DNA. Because each cell makes only certain proteins, only selected genes that encode for these proteins are active and copied into messenger RNA (mRNA) in a process called transcription.

While the DNA remains in the cell nucleus, the mRNA leaves the nucleus to instruct the cell as to what proteins to make in a process called translation, which takes place in the cytoplasm.

How does the cell know which genes need to be turned on and off at any given time? Transcription is regulated by specialized proteins called transcription factors, which either promotes (activators) or block (inhibitors) this process. These transcription factors respond to different cues from the cell environment to adjust the transcription rate of the required proteins.

For example, in healthy skin, very little collagen is being produced at any given time, and transcription inhibitors play the dominant role to keep collagen gene transcription turned off. However, during wound healing, collagen transcription is turned on because new collagen production is required to repair damaged tissue.

Once wound healing is completed, fibroblasts revert to their resting state and turn off collagen transcription. Increasing evidence now suggests that the process of transcription is disorderly in scleroderma fibroblasts.

Scleroderma fibroblasts produce excessive amounts of collagen protein because collagen transcription is increased. Many of the transcription activators and repressors involved in collagen regulation are already known, and it was found that scleroderma fibroblasts possess an excess of activators and diminished amounts of transcription inhibitors. These transcription activators and inhibitors are most likely also involved in the regulation of many other genes, beside collagen, that were found to be produced at abnormal levels by scleroderma fibroblasts.

Although transcription factors by themselves are not good therapeutic targets, because they are hidden inside the cells, this knowledge opens the door to other therapeutic potentials. As mentioned already, transcription factors respond to changes in the cell environment.

The signals from outside the cells are first received by specialized proteins on the cell surface called receptors and then relayed through the cytoplasm via a number of other specialized proteins called signal transducers into the nucleus. There, transcription factors respond to these signals by adjusting the transcription rate of specific genes.

Signal transduction pathways regulating collagen production are under intense study in many laboratories. Because signaling pathways are better therapeutic targets, this area of research should lead to the development of new treatments for scleroderma.

What causes the switch of scleroderma fibroblast to an activated state?

This still remains the least understood, but undoubtedly the most important area of scleroderma research. Because the switch occurs in the patient skin, most likely at a very early stage before any disease symptoms are apparent, it presents a great challenge to unravel the onset of the disease.

It is possible that other cells present in scleroderma lesions during the early stage of the disease send inappropriate signals to fibroblasts that permanently turns them on, resulting in excessive collagen production. An example of an activating signal is a factor secreted by immune cells termed Transforming Growth Factor-beta (TGF-beta).

TGF-beta is a potent inducer of collagen, and one theory suggests that it is responsible for the initial phase of the disease. However, why scleroderma fibroblasts remain turned on even in the absence of TGF-beta is still not well explained.

In trying to understand the causes of scleroderma, we must take into account other cells besides fibroblasts that may also behave abnormally in scleroderma lesions. For example, cells that line small blood vessels, called endothelial cells, become stressed and frequently die, causing damage to the vessel.

Although we do not know what causes these cells to die, their death may be directly connected to fibroblasts activation. Current studies are aimed at answering these remaining questions.

Future perspectives

The collective effort of many scientists dedicated to finding the cause and ultimately the cure for scleroderma has already uncovered many of the mysteries of scleroderma.

Patients contributing tissue biopsies used for research deserve special thanks. Without this generously donated material, most of the studies described in this article would not have been possible.

Because of the accelerated pace of scientific discoveries taking place today, and because scleroderma investigators are always on the cutting edge of new knowledge and technologies, we should be optimistic that the remaining questions will soon be answered and that the cure for scleroderma will be found in the near future.

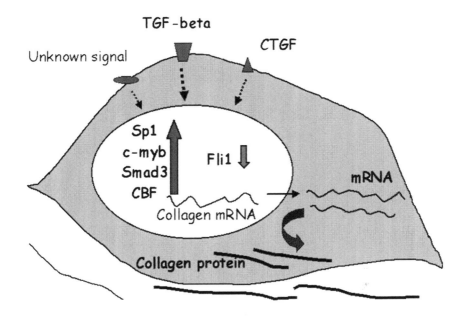

Diagram

In the scleroderma lesion, fibroblasts respond to outside signals that may originate from immune cells or other nearby cells. Current evidence points to TGF-beta and CTGF (connective tissue growth factor) as examples of signals involved in the activation of scleroderma fibroblasts, but not all of the signals are known.

These signals travel through specific cell surface receptors and intracellular signal transduction pathways (dashed lines) to their final destination in the cell nucleus where they are received by transcription factors. Many transcription activators such as Sp1, c-myb, Smad3 and CBF are unregulated, while a transcription inhibitor, termed Fli1, is diminished in scleroderma fibroblasts.

Together, these aberrations result in an increase in collagen gene transcription and mRNA synthesis. Collagen mRNA is then translated into collagen protein, which is secreted and deposited outside the cell.

In contrast, in healthy skin, fibroblasts are mainly at rest with only occasional collagen synthesis, which may be required for normal skin maintenance.

◆❖◆

Systemic Scleroderma Symptom Checklist

Please consult your doctor if you have two or more of the following symptoms, which are sometimes due to systemic sclerosis (scleroderma). Systemic scleroderma may disqualify a person for life and/or health insurance in some countries. Sometimes certain lab work or biopsy results may force an unwelcome diagnosis into the medical record.

Circulation
❑ Swelling of hands, feet and/or face
❑ Raynaud's: fingers and/or toes turn white or blue due to cold or stress
❑ Ulcers (sores) on fingertips or toes

Gastrointestinal
❑ Difficulty swallowing
❑ Heartburn (reflux)
❑ Constipation, diarrhea, irritable bowel syndrome

Heart, Lungs, Kidneys
❑ Shortness of breath
❑ Pulmonary (lung) fibrosis
❑ Aspiration pneumonia
❑ Pulmonary hypertension
❑ High blood pressure or kidney (renal) failure
❑ Right-sided heart failure

Muscles & Tendons
❑ Tendonitis, or carpal tunnel syndrome
❑ Muscle aches, weakness, joint pain

Excessive Dryness or Sjögren's Syndrome
❑ Excessive dryness of the mucus membranes (such as eyes, mouth, vagina), which is sometimes called Sjögren's Syndrome

Skin
❑ Tight skin, often on hands or face
❑ Calcinosis (calcium deposits)
❑ Telangiectasia (red dots on the hands or face)
❑ Mouth becomes smaller, lips develop deep grooves, eating and dental care become difficult

Many of these symptoms can occur by themselves or can be due to other things. Symptoms such as heartburn, high blood pressure, constipation, and muscle aches are very common in the general population. More unusual symptoms, such as tight skin and/or pulmonary fibrosis, may be more likely to lead to a scleroderma diagnosis.

◆ ❖ ◆

CHAPTER 2

Systemic Scleroderma
Caregiver Stories

*What do people do who are unfamiliar with
medical terms, insurance problems, and
changes in the disease process?*

—Betty J. Russo

Betty J. Russo
Husband, Systemic Scleroderma
California, USA

My husband was diagnosed with systemic scleroderma in November 2001. He had felt tired in August, and his hands became swollen in September. Then he developed sores on his fingertips in October.

It took two months to see a rheumatologist. He was put on a medication that made him very ill, so it had to be discontinued. He started a study medicine with the University of California in Los Angeles (UCLA), in September 2002, and so far here has not been a stop in the progression of his disease. It seems there is something new every week.

The latest is that he needs a special bed to prevent bed sores in the areas where his bones are not padded with normal tissue, since he has lost so much weight. He must take a laxative each week since his digestive system is slowing down. In the last two weeks we have obtained a wheelchair because he gets short of breath, a walker so he does not fall, a riser for the commode with arms so that he can get himself up, a seat in the shower because he cannot stand long enough to bathe, and a lift chair as he cannot get himself up anymore.

He cannot bathe, dress himself, or cut up his own food. He cannot wipe himself after using the toilet. This causes him great distress, for he was always so private about this. His skin is hard all over, his fingers are frozen almost closed, his legs are bent at the knees and hips and he cannot finish a can of soda because his head no longer flexes enough to drain the can.

He has been hospitalized with an infected joint in his finger requiring five days in the hospital and a month of home intravenous antibiotics, followed by oral antibiotics. After his HMO (managed care insurance) refused to pay for his brand of heartburn medication, he woke up with left arm pain and indigestion and had to go the emergency room. The diagnosis was esophageal spasm, and it could have been prevented by the right medication.

We are hoping that the study medicine will help, but it is hard to maintain hope since he continues to decline so fast. He lost a brother to scleroderma, but his brother lasted twenty years with it. The disease has been devastating for both of us, but the gyrations we must go through to receive decent medical care is almost as devastating. I am a registered nurse and I know the system, at least some of it.

What do people do who are unfamiliar with medical terms, insurance problems, and changes in the disease process? The lack of understanding, the constant problem solving with insurance coverage, the cold-shoulder care from physicians, and the daily process of enduring this disease has gotten to both of us. With the help of friends and family we will make it through. My heart and prayers go out to those who are suffering the same trials.

Cathy Bowell
Husband, Scleroderma
Ohio, USA

My husband, who is fifty-two years old, was diagnosed with sclero-derma in September 2000. Of course, it was quite a shock to hear what it actually was, but we had known something was wrong for several years because of the different symptoms he experienced.

I am thirty-seven years old and we are both confused about everything being thrown at us. I am trying to stay positive, but my husband is very pessimistic.

Update - August, 2002

Things are much better now. We have gotten through the last two years with all the support we have received from everyone at the www.sclero.org website.

The first year was the worst physically for my husband. He was on many different medications, and between the effects of the medications and the emotional strain, it was overpowering. Thankfully, my husband reacted positively to the medication and has been stable for eight months now.

I would love to hear from other spouses who would like to share their story. We are all here to support each other and get through this hard-to-understand disease together.

Thanks again for all the support and encouraging information you provide.

◆ ❖ ◆

Eliza
Mother-in-law, Morphea
Poland

This story was translated from Polish to English by Dr. Roy Smith and Dr. Magdalena Dziadzio. The original Polish Story can be found in Chapter 11.

Welcome. My name is Eliza and this story is not about me but about my mother-in-law.

Three years ago a mark appeared on her thigh. She thought she had hurt herself and that was the reason she had this blemish. After some time the mark started to grow bigger so she went to see a dermatologist, who took a biopsy.

Unfortunately, he did not make a clear diagnosis and started trial-and-error treatment; he also used steroids that were, however, not successful. Despite taking different tablets and applying various creams to the mark, no improvement was seen.

Later on, new marks appeared under one breast and in an armpit. My mother-in-law abandoned this doctor and went to see another one who also took a biopsy but then diagnosed scleroderma. The doctor said that the disease is incurable but not too severe; one has to learn how to live with it. And that is how he concluded his treatment.

In the meantime her ankle swelled up. She went to a rheumatologist who, after performing some tests, diagnosed lymphangitis and said that it could be linked to scleroderma.

The rheumatologist warned her that scleroderma is by no means a benign disease, but it can be linked to a stomach problem for which my mother-in-law has been treated for many years, as well as to her asthma. He concluded that scleroderma could attack the entire body including the bones and the internal organs.

Who should we listen to? Who is right? Where should we look for help?

To end, I add only that my mother-in-law has undergone several operations and has taken countless pills, but she is not an abuser of drugs.

Thank you for your interest.

◆❖◆

Janice
Mother, Scleroderma
Brazil

I am thirty-one years old and I live in Brazil. I decided to submit my story with the hope of getting more information about scleroderma. I have lupus and my mom has scleroderma. She is sixty-two years old and does not know that I am trying to understand her illness better.

I decided to do so because, although she pretends to be okay when she is near her children and grandchildren, my dad tells me all the time how sad she has been.

I do not know much about her symptoms because she hides them from me, but I can see how bad and ugly her skin is, especially her leg. One of her legs is much thinner than the other and she does not have strength in her legs, arms or hands anymore. She does not go swimming or wear Bermuda shorts because she is ashamed of her body.

I understand her in many ways, but I feel worried and sorry for her. Once dad told me she cried all night long because she had the impression the illness was getting to her internal organs.

I know how serious scleroderma is, but my question is: Will mom die soon? Will scleroderma get worse despite her treatment? Is there anything I can do to help her get better?

I have lupus, so I know how it feels to have a chronic illness. I think I understand her, but she is my mom and I do not want her to suffer like I do. I am afraid that scleroderma might be worse than lupus.

My mum has been getting worse although she tries to pretend she is better every time I call her and ask how she has been feeling. I usually call her three or four times a day to see how she is.

She has a lot of joint, muscle, and bone pain. It makes me feel miserable to see my dad carry her to the bathroom so she can brush her teeth. She has nausea all the time and I am not sure exactly what might be causing that. She has been going through many exams but we have not heard much from her doctor yet.

I hope I can help her somehow.

◆ ❖ ◆

Luis
Mother, Systemic Scleroderma
Spain

I would like to say that I believe my mother's illness was caused by the depression she suffered due to the death of my thirteen year old brother. Her nerves, depression and stress made her sick. The more depressed she became, the faster her scleroderma advanced on her hands and face.

But then, a will to live and to see her other sons grow struck her. At that moment, when her attitude changed from the path to death to the fight for life, her scleroderma stopped.

This is a message to all of those who are suffering or know of someone suffering with this rare illness. If you have passed through a big depression, try to do something that will distance yourself from being nervous, since it seems that helped stop the advance of scleroderma for my mother.

Mani
Mother, Systemic Scleroderma
India

My mother was always complaining of breathlessness, slight fever, and nails and fingers turning blue when exposed to cold air. This was more noticeable during winter when it was very cold.

She started developing frequent joint pain. She was given some pain-killers and advised to exercise regularly. The winter in Jalandhar lasts for four to five months and sometimes the temperature goes below freezing. But we ignored her complaints.

Next winter it happened again, and we continued to ignore it. We thought that it was due to fewer red blood cells. A couple of months later, in mid-1999, we were posted to Hyderabad and we noticed some white patches on the back of her neck. At first we thought that it was just due to a change in skin pigment, so we visited a general physician. He gave some ointment to be applied onto the skin, but it did not help.

We consulted another specialist in our town and after some inquiries, blood tests were done. When the specialist did not find anything, he asked for high resolution computed tomography (HRCT) of the lungs and this gave us the results of interstitial lung disease with honeycombing in the lower part of lungs.

My mother was offered steroids and she improved, but the dosage was not enough. Her body appeared swollen and we thought she was gaining weight, but she also complained of weakness and joint pain. Her physician increased the dosage.

Her life was easier after this. She would do everything, indoor as well as outdoor work, but on October 16, 2001, she got high fever that lasted for a week. The doctor referred her to a rheumatologist, but her condition was very bad and we were not able to visit the doctor.

October 27, 2001, is the day I will never forget. Her breathlessness was so bad that she was not able to talk, eat or drink, and she was immediately admitted to the intensive care unit.

The doctor was very nice. He told us the truth, that my mother had been diagnosed with a rare, incurable illness, systemic scleroderma with interstitial lung disease (ILD) and respiratory failure type-1. He told us that very little medication was known for helping it and that she would remain only on oxygen.

He was unable to tell us how long she would live. Her lungs were not working properly and the cause of it was also unknown, hence we were told that a cure was impossible. After listening to the doctor, we were totally shocked as we had never heard of such a disease and moreover we did not have any information or idea regarding systemic scleroderma.

My mother was prescribed many medications and she was told not to touch or hold anything cold. One medication caused her terrible side effects with red patches on her whole body, so the doctor discontinued it. Meanwhile, the white patches disappeared, never to be seen again.

Over the next few months she lost weight dramatically and was just a "bag of bones"! Sometimes she had swelling in her ankles and knees and pain in her joints.

Now my mother's condition is such that she cannot live without her oxygen concentrator. Her fingers are swollen, her face is tight, and her lips are drawn.

It is now affecting her hands and feet. She had some severe medication side effects the past few months. Her face started swelling, she gained a lot of weight and she started feeling pressure in her eyes, so her doctor reduced the dosage. For extreme pain in her chest we apply ointment and keep it covered with woolen clothes until she feels comfortable or painless. She is now taking six different medications.

I believe in miracles and know she will be healed soon. My message is: Have faith. Be strong! Do not give up! Face the reality and fight. Never lose hope.

◆ ❖ ◆

Sandra Joy Raumer
Husband, CREST
Washington, USA

I would first like to thank you for giving people the opportunity to tell their stories. It feels good to just unload!

My husband had all kinds of things happening to him that just did not seem right. We went to doctor after doctor, to emergency rooms, and finally to a rheumatologist, since these strange symptoms came upon him about three months ago.

At one of the emergency rooms, I asked the doctor to just take an educated guess. He said, "I think he has scleroderma."

Neither one of us had ever heard of scleroderma, so I asked the nurse to write it down for me. Then I started surfing the Web and came upon your wonderful Web site! I truly think if it had not been for you I would not have found out that my husband has CREST. I would really like to say that instead of second-guessing, we now know what he has so we can deal with it properly.

I would like all the patients out there to be persistent. Do not give up! You can deal with this. Trust me, if I can, you can too! There are medications out there which help the symptoms. We are just starting to find this entire thing out. I have found that my faith really helps me through this.

My husband asked, "Why is this happening to me?" Now we know why: it is so that we can share with others out there who suffer with this disease. I have personally cried rivers over this as I felt so useless. But now I know we must share with all of you. Please do not give up, be persistent, and share with others.

◆ ❖ ◆

Silvy
Sister, Scleroderma
Italy

My sister has had scleroderma for six years. Every day her physical aspect changes. At first, I accompanied her everywhere—to Rome, Palermo, Catania, to every hospital where they said they knew about scleroderma. Now she goes to the hospital a week every month to take a very strong medicine.

I was reading a lot about this illness, but now I am really feeling helpless because I feel powerless. I see my sister getting worse from day to day. She is thirty-five and has a son who is only six years old.

Her husband is always away and busy at work, and I work too. How can we take care of her? How do we defeat this terrible, fatal enemy? Please, help me discover a medicine, which could help her live as long as possible so that she will know her son's children.

I would like someone to give me addresses of hospitals, names of new medicines, and information on any new discoveries.

My sister was the most beautiful girl in our little village in Sicily. Now her skin is like wood, her mouth so little, and I cannot look at her hands without an escape to cry. Her fingers are deformed. She is embarrassed to enter into a shop to buy something and to hand them the money.

What happened to my sister?

Theresa
Mother, Diffuse Scleroderma with CREST
New York, USA

My mom, Mary, was diagnosed with diffuse scleroderma with CREST when she was only in her early twenties. She has now had it for over twenty years. At a very young age I was told that my mom suffered from a rare disease. So I told my mom that when I grew up I was going to become a doctor and find a cure for her.

As I got older I noticed slight changes in her appearance. Red spots began appearing on her face, neck, and hands. As time went on, she lost a lot of weight. She was always sick with sinus infections, pneumonia, and upper respiratory tract infections. She never tried to find a doctor that was familiar with this disease.

I went to BOCES nursing program while attending high school. I graduated in 2000, and I got my nursing license in 2002. After going to school, I found myself paying closer attention to her health. I noticed that she was having severe, uncontrollable fits of coughing and that she seemed to be having a hard time breathing. I asked one of the doctors I worked with whether they knew of any good physicians who had any experience with scleroderma. Luckily he gave me a name and my mom went to see him. After meeting the doctor she decided that she really liked him and switched doctors. He immediately did blood tests and sent her to a cardiologist, pulmonologist, and a scleroderma specialist.

Over the years we had all been in denial, ignoring the fact that we knew that she had a serious disease that can be fatal. Her visit to the specialist gave our whole family a reality check. The doctor said she may need a lung transplant if the damage to her left lung is as severe as he believes it is. That news was given to us over two weeks ago and it is just sinking in now.

On November 5, 2002, we will find out if she definitely needs the transplant. I know that I speak for my whole family when I say that we are nervous wrecks. My brother and I already told mom that if she does need the transplant that we want to be tested to see if we are a tissue match. That way if we are, she won't have to be put on a donor list. She doesn't like the idea of us doing that. Hopefully the doctor will give us good news. Until we find out, all we can do is pray.

◆❖◆

CHAPTER 3

Systemic Scleroderma
Patient Stories

She looked thoughtful for a moment,
and then quietly asked,
"Is there hope?"
—Gertie

Introduction
Finding New Ways to Cope
by Judith Thompson Devlin

Judith Thompson Devlin is Chair of the Archivist Committee for the International Scleroderma Network (ISN), and co-editor of this Voices of Scleroderma book series.

Life is full of daily events where we must tap into a myriad of coping mechanisms just to get through the day. Some coping methods are instinctual and feel more like a simple reaction to an incident. Some are learned behavior responses. However, if an event never experienced before happens, especially a health-related event, we are often clueless about how to deal with it.

We are seldom prepared for the diagnosis of a chronic incurable disease and it often leaves us feeling helpless as to how to handle this scary and unfortunate information and all the peripheral problems that come with the disease.

There are several emotional, physical and mental stages we go through during the coping process. In general the emotional stages are shock, numbness, fear, depression, panic, anger, hostility, apathy, denial, isolation and finally acceptance. Our physical coping methods depend on our individual symptoms and the physical limitations brought on by the disease. Mental coping is determined by how well we do with the emotional and physical coping.

Some of us get stuck in one stage and become unable to work through the other stages, with the final goal being acceptance. Some of us breeze through all the stages. However fast or slow we experience hearing the physician's words, "You have an incurable chronic and sometimes deadly disease," depends on how well we have learned to cope with life. No matter how quickly we travel through these stages, hearing these words from a physician can dramatically alter our sense of reality and overall stability.

Some of us will withdraw, isolate ourselves and live in a state of depression. Some will self-medicate with drugs and alcohol; some will whine and complain the rest of their days, some will pray, meditate and bargain, and others will find a new lease on life and try to live each moment as if it were our last.

Whatever coping mechanism we choose, it helps if we have family, friends, good and knowledgeable doctors and loving caregivers available to assist us when needed.

Some of us may feel abandoned by those we thought would always be there. Some of us will sense judgment by others or feel ignored and discarded. For whatever reason, in our society if a chronically ill person is not in a wheelchair, bedridden, bleeding or foaming at the mouth, we are often disbelieved.

We, the chronically ill, have more than our share of new problems to deal with, let alone coping with the disease itself. All of the ways we deal with illness is coping.

I have learned to see my scleroderma as a blessing in disguise. But before I got to this place, I experienced most of the stages mentioned above. I did seem to breeze through many of the stages soon after I was diagnosed because it was such a relief to know I was not crazy. I knew for years that something just was not right. I had many doctors pooh-pooh my complaints, minimize my symptoms and/or blamed my stressful lifestyle. Depression was a major problem for me for years, as was anger at myself for not feeling good.

Then once I was diagnosed and was told I had five to seven years left, I crammed a lot of living into that time period. But then the five to seven year time frame flew by. So yet another stage of coping presented itself with "What do I do now?".

I thought I had done all my living and had no regrets. I had made peace with everyone. My will was written. Now, I needed more coping skills. I had to make more plans. That was five years ago.

Life is funny, it just keeps happening. If not with us, it is happening all around us. So my credos kicked in big time: A day at a time; Don't let anyone waste my time; Stay away from negativity; Ignore the thoughtlessness of others; Be honest; Try not to take anything personally or make assumptions of other's actions, words and deeds and always try do my best.

For the most part I ignore my scleroderma, at least until it reminds me that I have overexerted, when I do not have energy and ache so bad I can barely move, or when I look in the mirror and see signs of it (although most of it could just be old age settling in.) Thinking this always makes me feel normal. And if I feel normal, I know it has been an okay day. That is acceptance. That is when I know I am coping. But tomorrow may be a bad day and another coping method may be required.

Coping is a daily event done mostly subconsciously. Every new symptom brings a new need for us to cope and find a better, easier way to do ordinary things. Sometimes we may have to stop a hobby, a job or a habit because we are no longer able to cope with it.

However, if we become more aware of coping skills and how we tend to use them, we can make better daily choices to cope and live with a more positive attitude and outlook on life in general. Sometimes just finding the humor in our plight and laughing at ourselves can be a great way to cope at any given moment.

It helps me a lot to read or hear the voices of how other chronically ill people cope. Many new or better coping mechanisms are related by sharing experiences. When we know that another is not coping well, we can extend a helping hand and it is usually appreciated.

The Voices of Scleroderma books serve well in this regard, as there are dozens of great coping stories. I hope that you, the reader, will find new ways to cope if you are having a difficult time; that you will admire the moxie and ingenuity of others, and find solace in the fact that indeed, life goes on, no matter what.

Debby B.
Systemic Scleroderma
Florida, USA

I was thirty-eight when I was diagnosed with scleroderma. That was two years ago, and since then my life has changed dramatically.

At the end of 1999, I began having unexplained aches and fatigue, as well as swelling and numbness in my hands. I suffer from Raynaud's, even though I live in a southern state where it is always warm.

My family has a history of autoimmune diseases, from rheumatoid arthritis to lupus, so I thought my Raynaud's was related to arthritis. My aunt had been diagnosed with lupus at a well-known clinic in our state, so I made an appointment there.

After a week of tests and a return trip a month later, I was given the diagnosis of scleroderma. The awful thing is, my first thought was, "Whew, at least it is not lupus." Little did I know. Once I realized what scleroderma involved, I was devastated.

Through a friend I found a wonderful rheumatologist who I now see every month. In the fall of 2000, I developed severe hypertension and my rheumatologist sent me to a nephrologist. He put me on medication, but my blood pressure stubbornly remained high.

In July 2001, everything came to a head. I was suffering from what I thought was a bad summer cold or sinus infection. I saw my family doctor, who prescribed an antibiotic and bed rest. Several days later I was worse. I had trouble breathing, bad headaches, a rapid heart beat, and nausea.

Finally, when I could barely get a breath, my husband rushed me to the hospital. My blood pressure when I arrived in the emergency room was 250/150. The doctors told my husband that I would have died if we had waited just five more minutes to come in. I had suffered congestive heart failure brought on by a renal hypertensive crisis. I spent three days in the intensive care unit and a week in the hospital until the doctors found the right combination of blood pressure medications.

To say that experience was an eye opener would be a major understatement. I have learned to take every cough, hive and symptom seriously. I bless every day that I am able to be up and around, walking, shopping for groceries, driving myself, taking care of our home, and all the little things we normally take for granted.

I do not know what is ahead of me, but who does? I try to stay positive and optimistic, otherwise my loved ones, my husband and family, just feel more helpless.

I pray for a cure in the very near future. I am lucky. I have a wonderfully supportive and understanding husband, a warm and loving family, and an excellent team of doctors who take extremely good care of me.

I cannot stress enough the importance of finding compassionate physicians who are knowledgeable about scleroderma. I am not giving up. I plan on being around for a long time.

Donna S.
Systemic Scleroderma
Tennessee, USA

I am a thirty-nine year old female. I suffered my first symptoms in May 1999, and was diagnosed in October 1999. I have systemic scleroderma.

The major involvement is in my ankles and feet. I have joint stiffness in my fingers, hands, wrists, and knees even though I don't have any skin hardening in those areas.

I have skin hardening on my ankles and the top of my feet. My toes are fine. I do not have any internal organ involvement yet.

I also do not have Raynaud's and I have no problem with cold temperatures, other than a slight stiffness in my joints. I have never had ulcers on my fingers or toes. I have never had internal organ involvement, so I am not text-book systemic.

My dermatologist has spoken with many dermatologists across the country, and they have not heard of my particular type of scleroderma. They also have not heard of blisters being associated with scleroderma in any form, but I certainly have them.

My first symptoms started as muscle fatigue and soreness. Then I retained a lot of fluid all over. I was given medication to relieve the fluid, which worked quite well. I lost six pounds of fluid the first night I took it.

Soon after that my hands began to draw up. I had four months of physical therapy and now I am able to completely open my hand and make a fist, although I still have some joint contractures.

I had begun light treatment for three months, but I had to stop the treatment due to ulcers forming on my ankles, in July 2000. I was forced to take a leave from work as a result of this and I was confined to a wheelchair. I used Unna Boots and numerous creams, and finally in January 2001, the ulcers healed.

I filed for disability through my employer and Social Security, and was denied by both. I then began five months of physical therapy on my knees, ankles, and toes. I responded well to this therapy, and I was able to return to work in July 2001. I worked part time in July, and then I began full time in August.

Later that month I began to have severe itching on my ankles. My dermatologist prescribed hydrocortisone cream for it. After using the cream for about a week, I developed a large blister on my right ankle. I thought this was an allergic reaction to the medication so I discontinued it. My physical therapist stopped my therapy because she did not want me to tear the skin off the blister.

Soon after, more blisters developed. They are very large, sometimes covering the entire side of my ankle, and they are very painful. I have visited the University of Virginia Medical School in Charlottesville and my dermatologist, and they have never seen this condition with scleroderma, nor do they have a solution for it. I have tried megadoses of prednisone, numerous ointments and creams, and elevation of my ankles, but nothing has helped.

It has now been a year since these blisters started, and they are still going strong. I had to leave work in March 2002, and I have finally received my Social Security disability benefits, but I have to be reviewed in May 2003 for continued benefits. I have applied for long-term disability benefits through my employer, although it has not been approved yet.

I am thankful that I do not have internal organ involvement, but these blisters are really taking their toll on me, with continual pain. I get to the point sometimes when I don't even think I will survive.

I am hoping that someday someone finds a cure for this dreadful disease, but until then, I, like you, will continue to suffer.

◆ ❖ ◆

Gertie
Systemic Scleroderma
California, USA

Early in 2001, it hit me that since childhood I have had numerous inflammatory conditions, many of which are chronic and lifetime such as dermatitis, gingivitis and more. I had developed allergies in adolescence. During my only pregnancy I was virulently nauseous. I threw up constantly until medicated, causing my doctor to comment that it seemed I might be allergic to pregnancy hormones. It seems to me that some kind of inflammation or self-rejection process was always going on.

Then in February 2001, the possible engine driving this inflammation process fully manifested itself in what I now call my year of total health meltdown. I had started a challenging new job and within a month I developed increasingly severe swelling in my hands, arms, feet and legs.

At night I would awaken with my right hand asleep or with a stabbing pain in my left upper arm, or with a strange tingling sensation running up my leg, or a sharp burning pain in my toe.

I had had several of these symptoms for about four years, but they were becoming more urgent and troubling. My feet were so swollen and painful that I had to wear soft clogs to work.

I saw my general practitioner for the toe pain and she diagnosed osteoarthritis, but I knew it was not that. I had felt a change in my system the preceding autumn, like a change of gears in a car, as if I was coming down with something.

My eyes had begun to water profusely when I was outdoors, and I got tired faster. My doctor did a blood test and my antinuclear antibody (ANA) was 1:80, which was borderline positive, and it was in the nucleolar pattern. She insisted my pain was arthritis. As the symptoms intensified, I asked her for a referral to a rheumatologist.

The next six months became a blur of pain, uncertainty, anxiety and tests. I kept wondering when I could just take a pill and it would all go away. They monitored my blood, urine, neurology and all my major organs. I had magnetic resonance imaging (MRI), CT scans, pulmonary function test (PFT), ultrasounds, and twenty-four hour urine tests. All this testing intensified my anxiety, which I think was fueling the underlying condition and the inflammation in my hands and feet.

My health meltdown continued. I was diagnosed with hiatal hernia after I complained of heartburn and food getting caught in my throat. I developed persistent moderate asthma and had to begin using inhalers. I kept my rheumatologist informed of these health developments, and in about six months, a complete picture began to emerge.

After an EMG to try to determine a neurological cause for the leg tingling, the neurologist said there was no neurological problem, but that I probably had a serious connective tissue disease called lupus. My rheumatologist had been doing tests all along to exclude lupus.

I finally asked her bluntly what, if anything, I had. She told me I was in the early stages of an autoimmune disease that is a cousin of lupus. That stung. Insurance companies do not like things like lupus or its family members. So we tacitly agreed that we would not hang labels on the aches and pains we discuss.

Due to the economic depression, I lost my job in August, which was a blessing. I could not control the swelling, and had some very tough days. Heavy fatigue, mind fog, and pain had crowded out my productivity.

Then on September 12, 2001, as the television in the background re-played the horrific scenes of the 9/11 tragedy, I learned about scleroderma from my Internet research and from a book by Dr. Maureen Mayes.

The only connective tissue disease whose early stages are swollen hands and feet and that is a cousin of lupus became clear: scleroderma sans scleroderma or systemic sclerosis without skin involvement.

Then I understood why my rheumatologist always pinched my skin, and aggressively monitored every major organ function and my rising blood pressure. She asked repeatedly if my hands and feet ever got cold and if I could swallow okay, and told me to go to the emergency room if I devel-oped certain symptoms.

In September my ANA was higher than 1:650, which my rheuma-tologist called "through the stratosphere," and it was in a pattern strongly associated with scleroderma.

I stopped taking one medication in October because it was raising my blood pressure. In November I went to the emergency room with acute stomach pain and vomiting and they did an upper abdominal CT scan. The problem was probably a virus, but the technician reported a scar on the base of my lung. When I told my rheumatologist about this, she jumped to the computer and pulled down the technician's report. I ended up getting another CT of my lung within weeks. Luckily, it was inconclusive, and we will retest in six months.

In January of 2002, I asked for medication for anxiety, and cutting off my constant anxiety was like turning off the aggressive progression of this disease. Without working, my stress level has decreased. Stress and anxiety seem to be triggers of my disease. By February my rheumatologist said my disease had stabilized and my swelling had greatly subsided. I asked her what I might expect next, and she shrugged her shoulders saying, "It is what it is."

For the past two weeks I have been doing a home renovation project, and my condition has destabilized. My hands are again swollen with soft tissue pain, and I have arthralgic pain in my right pinkie. My hand fell asleep last night, waking me up so I had to shake it.

I still have no signs of Raynaud's, although I do have a migraine condition. I do not have any skin thickening or hardening, either. But my hair is falling out again, my asthma is worsening, and my right hand feels like a tight old leather glove and is red hot.

It has taken several months for me to come to any terms of acceptance, and I avoid thinking of my condition by name. Denial, anger, grief and frustration all converge at once.

Some of my family members say I am a hypochondriac and they tell me to stop reading the medical encyclopedia. My husband is strangely skeptical, which I interpret as his form of denial. My sister sides with his challenging attitude, saying it is all in my head.

But my friends understand and have been very supportive and sympathetic. Above all, my mother understands. She asked me a very poignant question after I explained the illness to her. She looked thoughtful for a moment, and then quietly asked, "Is there hope?"

Her simple question forced me to arrive at a conclusion after all the things I had researched about scleroderma. In an instant I reviewed all I had read of the suffering and disability and the statistics and the cold clinical details in medical journal articles. Well, is there hope? After some thought, I told her, "Yes." Her smile brightened my day.

◆❖◆

James F. Hickey
Systemic Scleroderma
New York, USA

I am fifty-eight years old and until four years ago, I was the picture of health. Then on Father's Day morning I was painting the trim of my house when I fell from the ladder, breaking my ankle and spraining my neck.

After surgery I went through rehabilitation, and was forced to retire from my position. I owned a small food brokerage business in central New York. The standing, driving, and lifting were beyond my new limitations, and I was taking painkillers.

Shortly after rehabilitation, I started having some predictable problems, including arthritis and a few bad reactions to medications. I noticed swelling in my hands and visited the first of many doctors about this. First they said it was Lyme disease, then rheumatoid arthritis, and then, almost a year later, scleroderma. Strangely, that was just the beginning of my problems.

I have a disability policy that is supposed to take care of me for life if I am forced to retire due to an accident. My policy has been in effect for the last three years. This week two representatives of the company visited me with some disturbing news. To their thinking, now that I have scleroderma they should be off the hook, because my policy covers accidents and not disease.

I called my doctor, who supports my claim that my ankle is never going to repair itself, either with or without scleroderma. However, I will have to put up with a full hearing before the insurance company in order to keep my benefits. I know this is just a ploy to get me to settle. I have already been found fully disabled by Social Security for my ankle alone, but this is not enough for the folks at the insurance company. I will have to hire a lawyer at my own expense to keep the benefits.

I am sure this is just the start, and that they will never leave me alone. The only thing every doctor I have visited has told me is to avoid stress. As most of us know, stress causes flare-ups and things always hurt just a little more. The lesson I have learned is to *never* believe an insurance company.

◆❖◆

Kath
Systemic Scleroderma
Spain

I am Scottish, but I recently moved to Spain for the much warmer climate. I lived in northeast Scotland in the city of Aberdeen until just over a year ago. Moving to Spain has had a positive effect on my Raynaud's, but no effect on my scleroderma.

I have suffered with Raynaud's for thirty years. Thirteen years ago, it was discovered that I also had systemic sclerosis (scleroderma).

I believe my illness began when I was eighteen, when I developed allergies after I became pregnant with my daughter. The condition worsened after my son was born two years later, when I developed asthma. It was a few years after that when my Raynaud's was diagnosed. I have had poor health since then, always going to the doctor with some problem or another.

I suffered from a lot of stress with a two bad marriages that ended in divorce. I finally married a loving, caring and supportive man, but my health problems continued.

When I was thirty-seven, I was sent for tests at a local skin clinic. At last I had a name for what was wrong with me: systemic sclerosis. It was not all in my mind after all!

I joined the Scleroderma and Raynaud's Association in the United Kingdom, and through them I learned a lot about scleroderma. I was a patient at Ninewells Hospital in Dundee, Scotland, under Professor Belch, for nine years and during that time I had regular monitoring of the disease.

I still need to find a specialist here in Spain. I am fifty now and have recently taken early retirement from my work, due to ill health. I have often suffered from stress, and family and work-related problems have only added to that.

I have many symptoms associated with scleroderma, including high blood pressure and high cholesterol, despite trying not to eat animal fat. I have an underactive thyroid, and dry eyes and mouth. I take many medications, but I am determined not to let the illness take over my life.

I am studying the Spanish language and culture, and I still look forward to new activities and challenges. My husband has a work contract here in Spain and we both want to continue to stay here in this wonderful sunny climate.

I believe my problems began with pregnancy, although there is no scientific proof of that. The experts say that chemical exposures sometimes cause scleroderma, but I don't think I have been exposed to any such chemicals.

However, I have had a lot of stress, and that could be a contributing factor. Nobody in my family has scleroderma, although asthma, heart and kidney disease, high blood pressure and high cholesterol certainly runs in my family.

I don't think my family really understands my condition and what affect it has on my life, but my husband has always been very supportive.

Scleroderma is difficult for any of us to understand as the symptoms vary from person to person. I hope there is an answer out there for us all.

Lynn S.
Systemic Scleroderma
North Carolina, USA

I will be twenty-eight in a few weeks. My story started about seven years ago. I had a spot on my arm that was diagnosed as morphea.

A few years ago, I started having problems with my left arm and shoulder hurting. After about five tests the doctors decided it must be tendonitis. Now my neck hurts all the time. I also have tendonitis in my left Achilles tendon.

I had reflux for years, and then it started feeling like there was something stuck in my throat all the time. The muscles in my esophagus will not relax, so I take muscle relaxers plus pills for reflux. I also have Raynaud's, seronegative arthritis, and myositis.

A few weeks ago, I found out that I have mild pulmonary hypertension, so I am being sent to a specialist. It took many tests before they figured that out. I have a lot of pain and am very tired. I have trouble climbing stairs and hills.

It was not easy getting to the root of my problems. Most of the doctors I had seen thought I was full of it. No one believed me, I guess because I look healthy. I would always hear, "You are too young for this!"

I credit my pulmonary doctor for my diagnosis, as he kept looking into my breathing problem. It may have taken six tests, but he finally did get to the bottom of it.

I do not know what I will feel like in five or ten years, but for now I get up and go to work every day. My family has been very good. My mother always believed me and my sister, who is a nurse, did too.

I don't think my husband realizes how much pain I am in all the time, but overall, he understands. We have only been married for about two years and would really like to have a child, so I will be consulting my doctors to see if pregnancy is advisable or not, given my health situation.

I am very glad there are people here who understand.

◆ ❖ ◆

Maria
Systemic Scleroderma
Ukraine

This story was written by Maria in English and translated back into Russian by Dr. Alexandra Balbir-Gurman. The Russian translation can be found in Chapter 12.

I am fifty years old, and I was born in the Ukraine, a country where winter is very cold. I was a healthy child. I liked snow and frost. I ran in the snow, rode sleds, and made yeti (snowmen). I did not freeze and I was very happy.

What is happening with my hands now? They do not endure any cold. Their color varies from white to dark blue, and I cannot move my fingers very well. This began fifteen years ago, and my doctor says it is Raynaud's disease.

When my struggle began, I accepted a lot of medicine, but my illness still progressed. Dark stains and ulcers formed on my fingers.

I live in a small town and in a poor country. My doctors have no computers or medical journals. I went to a medical center to see a rheumatologist, and she has helped me very much. She said I have scleroderma, and she prescribed medications for me.

The wounds on my fingers have disappeared, but other symptoms have begun. I have grown very thin, so my clothes have become too large for me. I have lost eleven kilograms (twenty-five pounds) during the last two years. My friends ask me how I manage to have such a good figure. They do not know that I have been getting injections of anabolic steroids.

My muscles have become so thin that I cannot sit on a rigid chair, so I have put soft pillows on all the chairs in my room. Now I compete with my cat (who is faster) as to which of us will occupy a soft chair first.

When I began searching on the Internet for a treatment, I found this www.sclero.org Web site. But this created a new problem for me, as the information was in English! What should I do? I studied English many years ago, so I decided not to despair. I am unable to read the text from the screen, so I printed it out on paper. Then I took a big dictionary and I slowly began to translate it.

I say many thanks to Shelley Ensz and to everyone else who has made this Web site. I have begun to learn a lot of new things. I want to cure my illness. I ask all doctors to help me! I shall wait for your advice!

I am a teacher, so I work at a school. I feel numbness in my hands so I cannot hold a piece of chalk. I try to hide my ill hands from my pupils.

My husband advises me to remain at home, but I want to go to work. When I come onto the school courtyard, the pupils run to me and cry to me, "Good morning!" Then I have no time to think about illness. I smile to them and I answer, "Good morning!" It is my salvation.

I want to have friends with the same illness as me.

Sheena R.
Systemic Scleroderma
North Carolina, USA

My symptoms began about three years ago, however; thinking back, they may have begun even before that. I had always been a fast-paced, high-strung, typical type-A person, so I knew something was wrong when it began to take every ounce of energy I could muster just to get out of bed.

I went to see my longtime family doctor with flu-like symptoms. The routine blood work was drawn, and I was told to take a few days off to rest. The next morning my doctor referred me to a hematologist because I was severely anemic.

I had been a registered nurse for ten years and could not believe I had lost that much blood without noticing it. So the nightmare began. After two blood transfusions, four endoscopies and colonoscopies, and lots of money, I was diagnosed with watermelon stomach (WS). The diagnosis took two years. By then my family and I were pretty disheartened.

I was convinced I would die before anyone decided how to help me. My fingers became swollen and turned blue when they were exposed to cold. I was often bloated, never seemed to eat, and began to notice changes in my bowel habits. I had fatigue and I just plain felt bad all the time, but I still continued to believe I was cured after each laser treatment on my stomach. None of my doctors could understand how all my other complaints went along with the watermelon stomach, but I knew they did!

Finally, my hematologist decided to find out why my antinuclear antibody (ANA) titer was always high and he referred me to a rheumatologist. Three and a half years after my first symptoms, I was officially told I had scleroderma and that there was no cure, and that the best I could hope for was treatment for my symptoms. That was six months ago. Since then I have gone for a second opinion at the urging of my family, and have started more medications.

I also have developed moderate pulmonary hypertension, so I will need echocardiograms every two months for the rest of my life to monitor it.

My story is not very different from many others I have read over the past few months, but I feel like I need to share it with people who could really understand how this disease changed my life. It cannot be compared to any other illness that I can think of. At least with cancer, you can some idea what to expect.

I am fortunate as I am forty years old and have raised five children. My youngest child is eighteen, and I have two wonderful grandchildren whom I adore. I only wish I still had the energy in my body that my mind and heart still possess.

Seema Naqvi
Systemic Scleroderma
India

I am a forty-three year old Indian Hindu mother of two daughters, who are twelve and seven. My first symptoms began in 1993, three years after my first delivery, with clubbing of my fingers. No physician could tell me the cause. One doctor identified it as early scleroderma and prescribed some medications, but I was scared of the possible side effects, so I did not take them.

At the end of 1993, I suddenly began to have severe bouts of dry coughing. Each bout lasted for thirty to forty minutes. Doctors found fibrosis in my lungs.

At the same time, I got pregnant. One physician advised me to terminate the pregnancy and start a medication, but I refused. However, my gynecologist encouraged me to continue the pregnancy, and closely monitored the fetal growth. Miraculously, all of my symptoms vanished while I was pregnant.

I gave birth to my second daughter in September 1995. She is absolutely normal and tops her grades in school. During lactation, I did not have any cough, only the clubbing with Raynaud's. However, when I stopped breast feeding in June 1997, the cough started again. The bouts were shorter than before, but gradually their duration and frequency increased.

All this while, I was running from one doctor to another and had numerous test. Finally I came to know about Dr. V. R. Joshi, an internist who specializes in rheumatic diseases. He started treatments that stopped the deterioratoin of my lungs. I still had shortness of breath, but no coughing bouts. Then during the winter months of November and December in India, my lung problem was aggravated.

My real woes started in January 2002, when I developed severe arthritis. My fingers became swollen and my knee joints became inflamed. The soles of my feet hurt like hell. My doctor changed my medications, and now I only feel better when the anti-inflammatory drug is working.

I have left my fate to God. I am confident that I will survive with His blessings.

❖❖❖

Tony B.
Systemic Scleroderma
Ohio, USA

I was diagnosed with scleroderma in September of 2000, but I had the symptoms for three years before that.

I am sure I do not have to tell any of you what it felt like to be told I had scleroderma and a poor prognosis. It has taken me some time to come to terms with this disease. The ISN website and the support of others who have scleroderma has helped me tremendously.

When I was diagnosed with scleroderma through blood work, I was sent to a local rheumatologist who started me on medications with a wait-and-see attitude.

I live one hour from the Cleveland Clinic in Ohio, which is one of the best clinics in the country. I found a good rheumatologist who dove right into the problem by scheduling breathing tests, lung scans, heart tests and complete blood work.

I found out I have Raynaud's (which I already knew), pulmonary fibrosis and pulmonary hypertension. About thirty percent of my lungs had scar tissue so I was put on chemotherapy and an antibiotic to stop the lungs from scarring more. He also started me on blood pressure medication to treat the Raynaud's.

After I was on chemotherapy for about a year, I had another lung scan which showed that the scarring had stopped. Today I am doing better than two years ago and I am pretty much stable on my medications. However, I am still limited with what I can do because of the scarring of my lungs and the shortness of breath.

I still have a lot of pain throughout my body, with more severe pain in my fingers and hands, and all the rest that goes along with scleroderma.

◆ ❖ ◆

Valerie Holmes
Systemic Scleroderma
Missouri, USA

I was diagnosed with systemic scleroderma on my birthday in June 2001. What a present!

Scleroderma, what is it? I still don't know for sure. I only know that since I have been labeled with it, my life has changed drastically.

Once diagnosed, I had to begin taking a regimen of drugs, and the effects made it necessary for me to take a two week leave from my job.

When my employer found out that I have scleroderma, he changed my job. When I went back to work, I was told that I no longer had my job, as it had been given to someone else.

People acted as if they were afraid of me. Even my closest friends and family were not sure how to treat me. Why? So far I do not look or act any different. I think people are afraid of me because they do not know what scleroderma is. I know the feeling, since I am afraid to find out too much about it, yet I still wonder what is going to happen to me next.

I have scleroderma in my esophagus, and it causes me to vomit a lot. My skin is getting tighter and my hands hurt. I feel tired, and I hate taking all of the medications.

Why so many drugs? They tell me it is to slow the disease down, but how do they know if the scleroderma is slowing down? It seems as though it is gradually getting worse, but I am not sure.

My husband seems to have very mixed emotions about how to handle my disease. He tries to keep me upbeat, and he does not like to hear about the pain and how I am feeling. He says that all I think of is the disease and when I am going to die.

◆❖◆

Annette L. Ditzler
Diffuse Scleroderma
Illinois, USA

I have read many of these stories and cried many tears over them. I feel so bad for everyone who suffers from this. Up until now, I have done very well at pretending not to be ill.

I was first diagnosed in 1984, when I was twenty-five years old, after the birth of my second child. But looking back, Raynaud's and leg cramps began when I was fifteen. I had been to doctors many times with what they termed "vague complaints" and was told I was too young and healthy to be having joint pain, chest pain, bowel difficulties, and so forth. They thought I was a hypochondriac and needed psychological help, so I decided to keep the pain to myself.

One day I developed red blotches with awful itching and burning on my face, arms, chest and legs. My left arm and hand swelled to three times its normal size, turned black, and was severely painful. Little ulcers formed on my fingertips.

I was sent to a rheumatologist, where I was diagnosed. I went through several doctors as they all seemed to take better jobs elsewhere, and I got very tired of having to repeat everything over again with each new doctor.

I was prescribed many different drugs and had adverse or allergic reactions to them. I was told over and over again to avoid cold and stress, and to quit smoking and coffee.

I graduated from nursing school in 1991 and visited my last physician in 1992. I am now forty-two years old, the mother of six children, and a self-employed Registered Nurse Consultant.

I have joined an exercise class to see if it will provide a miracle for my body. I was given approximately fifteen years to live from my diagnosis in 1984, and here I am seventeen years later. I chalk it up to stubbornness and avoidance of doctors. They may be great in all other fields, but not with scleroderma. I feel let down.

I alternate between different over-the-counter pain relievers, diuretics and laxatives, which I use conservatively. I tolerate as much pain as possible before using any medicine, but I do not push the pain to the point of injury.

I am getting tired of dealing with the widespread pain; the purple, cold, and clumsy hands; the numbness, pain and tingling in all extremities; the constipation, diarrhea and abdominal pain; the chest pain, flutters, palpitations and shortness of breath; the extreme weakness and fatigue; the fluid retention in my legs, hands and face; the severe itching and burning of my skin from head to toe; and the periods of insomnia. I also have a prolapsed mitral valve and sclerosing of the lining around the heart.

But the hardest thing for me to handle is the people who do not or cannot truly understand what I am going through. Or those who look at my hands when I am writing out a check in the store and say something like, "What is wrong with you? Your hands are purple!"

I try to keep it all to myself, because I think that if I speak about how I feel, it will get worse, and I would sound like a hypochondriac.

I push myself to try to do everything like I used to, and I get very frustrated when I cannot! But I am afraid if I give in and lay down, then I will truly die.

I do not want to be a burden to my family and that concerns me a lot. I feel guilty for placing this uncertain future burden upon them. I am thankful for all that I have and pray that I will be able to take care of all my children until they are out on their own. My baby is five.

If there are any new groundbreaking therapies, I may listen, but I am scared. There, now I said it. Thank you for letting me vent. I guess it has been building up in me for a long, long time.

◆ ❖ ◆

Annette Turner
Diffuse Scleroderma
Illinois, USA

I found out I had scleroderma on March 11, 2002. I had no idea what I had, I just knew there was something wrong. I liked it better when I did not know, because the more I learn about it, the more I worry.

I am thirty-seven years old. I have three wonderful children. Two of them are married and on their own. My fourteen year old is still at home and is a big help to me. I also have a wonderful granddaughter.

I have worked in jobs from nursing homes to factories since I was eighteen years old, up until last July, when I could not take the pain any longer.

I have had three surgeries. The first was on my right hand for carpal tunnel in March 2000. The second was on my left hand in April 2000. Then in July 2000, they did a right lateral elbow release, which helped for about a year until the pain returned. I just thought the surgeries had not been done right. Then my knees began constantly hurting.

I started having heartburn at night so bad that it felt like I was having a heart attack. My arms felt swollen, from my skin getting harder. My skin was getting darker all the time, and it looked as though I had been tanning. My face got harder, and my fingers were swollen, and it became harder and harder for me to use my hands.

I finally decided to see a doctor. On my first visit, he asked how I was doing. I told him I wasn't doing good or I wouldn't be there. He asked what he could do for me. I said I just needed him to listen, and I told him about everything that was happening.

Then he told me about scleroderma. I didn't really understand what he was telling me. He made an appointment for me to see a rheumatologist the next week. He also said I could look up scleroderma on the Internet and I would learn a lot more. That is how I found this site and read everything I could. I was scared to death to find out for sure I had this.

The rheumatologist sent me to the hospital for lab work, chest X ray, EKG, urinalysis and esophageal swallow. He said I had Raynaud's and scleroderma. He put me on a lot of medications, took me off work, and told me to sign up for disability.

Now I have lab work done every month. I see the doctor again in six weeks. He said that so far I just have hardening of the skin on my face, arms, hands, and neck. The hardening is only in my skin and not in my muscles, but it could go there, too.

My skin is shiny from head to toe. My mouth is getting so tight that I have trouble opening it wide enough to eat, and I have cuts on both sides of my mouth from opening it to eat. My internal organs are not affected yet.

I have lost all mobility in my hands. At night I cannot move my knees and hips because of the pain. My doctor said that is because the arthritis is really bad in my joints. After I have been sitting or lying too long in one spot, it is difficult and painful to stand up. I also have rheumatoid arthritis.

I have found this site very helpful in answering a lot of questions. I can see where having friends who understand what I am going through would be a big help. Most people think I look okay. They do not understand that I am hurting on the inside so much more than the eye can see.

Update – April 2003

On April 18, 2003, I went to see Dr. Richard Burt in Northwestern Memorial Hospital in Chicago. He explained the two different types of stem cell transplants, autologus and allogenic.

With an autologus transplant, they would harvest my own stem cells and try to reboot my immune system in order to reverse the effect of this disease. This carries less risk than an allogenic transplant, but since they would be using my own stem cells, there is less chance for remission or reversal of my illness.

With an allogenic transplant, they would test my siblings to find the best match. This is riskier, since my body could reject the donor blood, however there are medications that can reduce the risk of rejection.

My immune system would then take on the healthy immune system of my sibling donor, and this might possibly cure me. I have four sisters and an older brother, and they are all willing to be tested to see if they would be a good donor. I am going to have this procedure, even if they have to use my own stem cells.

I will stay in Chicago for some time in order for them to monitor my progress. I will be in isolation for awhile since they will give me chemo-therapy to kill my immune system. My sibling donor will also have to stay in Chicago for a short time to provide the stem cells. The risks to the donor will be minimal.

Anyway, all of this will be expensive. I will have to get a room or efficiency apartment close to the hospital to be accessible for the doctors to monitor me once I'm released from the hospital after the transplant.

I am going to call the Red Cross to see if the army will let my son Raymond, who is at war, come home so he can be here with me.

I hope for a good outcome for myself. If not, then I hope they learn a lot from it, which will help the next person. I will try to update my story as soon as I am able.

Christine Sim
Diffuse Scleroderma
Australia

I have diffuse stage 2 scleroderma. I was diagnosed in 1994, but I was having some symptoms in the early 1980s, when I told my doctor several times that my hands kept swelling, but all to no avail. It was not until December 1993, when my hands were terribly swollen and on fire, that I managed to get a reaction.

Soon thereafter, I had many tests by rheumatologists, neurologists, and dermatologists. Finally I was waiting for the psychiatrist! In my final visit with my first rheumatologist, he virtually told me to go home and get on with my life!

The shocked look on my face prompted him to suggest that I could seek a second opinion, if I wanted. In his defense, I should point out that at this stage my fingers had not yet started curling.

I grabbed this alternative with both hands and I have been with my terrific new rheumatologist for seven and a half years. My first visit with her brought the first mention of the "S" word, and three months later this diagnosis was confirmed.

I did not know whether to break out the tissues or the champagne or both! I was so happy that someone had finally agreed there was something wrong with me and that it had a name. She told me not to go reading medical books, but right away I went to the library and starting poring over and photocopying medical tomes.

I have had countless tests, including CAT scans, bone scans, X rays, blood and urine tests, lung function tests, ultrasounds, a HIDA scan, echocardiograms, lung scans, and MRI. I had a fibroid adenoma removed from my breast, an abdominal hysterectomy and oopherectomy, a colonoscopy, several gastroscopies, laser surgeries to my stomach, a prostacyclin infusion, a blood transfusion, iron infusions, finger surgeries, joint aspirations, a laparotomy, drainage of an ovarian cysts, and cortisone injections.

I also have a sizable list of medications. It makes first visits to new doctors and hospital check-ins a nightmare when it comes to recording and remembering my medical history! Besides, they never have enough room on the forms, so I made a list of the essentials on the computer and take copies of it with me when I go on any of these little sojourns. I also have a copy on hand at home in the event of an emergency.

Radiographers, pathology nurses and receptionists have all become familiar faces and greet me by name on sight, perhaps partly because I donate *National Geographic* magazines to their waiting rooms.

My husband is away a great deal with business, but I am always assured of his loving care whether he is at home or thousands of miles away. I have three wonderfully helpful and supportive daughters who are still at home, plus marvelous parents and in-laws close by. I also have excellent, patient and understanding doctors, including my rheumatologist, general practitioner and gastroenterologist.

I have always enjoyed knitting, sewing, and crocheting, but now my hands are not as dexterous, so now I do cross-stitch and ribbon embroidery. I have also discovered a passion for card making, which I am trying to turn into a bit of a money-spinner. I love gardening, too, but I need more help from my "apprentices" now.

Life certainly has its challenges. It seems a new one crops up every week! Despite several times when I have muttered between gritted teeth, "I do not want to be here anymore," I really wouldn't miss it for quids!

Darlene
Diffuse Scleroderma
Delaware, USA

In February of 1999, I fell while taking my four children skating. I thought that I might have fractured my right leg because I could not walk on it for a long time.

My primary care physician sent me for X rays, noticed my swollen hands, and ordered some blood tests. A few days later she called and told me that my X rays were fine, but that I had scleroderma. I had never heard of scleroderma before, and she was rather vague about it.

The first thing she said was, "Do not go on the Internet." So, the first thing I did was go online to see what it was. The more I read, the more I cried. My husband was convinced that I was going to die.

The most difficult part was trying to tell my mother. After being diagnosed for certain by my rheumatologist, I had to ask my older sister to explain it to mom because I was so upset that I could not talk for two days.

My rheumatologist sent me to a gastrointestinal specialist and a pulmonologist. The gastrointestinal specialist explained that sometimes people with scleroderma get throat cancer and suggested that I have an upper GI test performed, which only showed a few polyps.

The pulmonologist ordered a pulmonary function test (PFT) and found that I have some lung involvement. I had an exercise echocardiogram that showed I have mild pulmonary hypertension. After doing a monitored exercise program for eight weeks, my exercise echocardiogram improved.

Every month I have blood tests to make sure my medications are not interfering with my kidneys, and that is usually painful because my veins are so small.

I take fifteen pills a day to cope with all my symptoms from CREST, Sjögren's, rheumatoid arthritis, and pulmonary hypertension. I have skin tightening, acid reflux, fatigue, nausea, vomiting, swollen ankles and knees, and soreness all over.

Some days I cry and am very depressed, but I joined a support group and that has helped me cope with scleroderma. I think I have one of the most supportive husbands in the world and I do not think I would be sane without him. My siblings have also been very supportive and they call to check on me often.

Now that I have become more knowledgeable about scleroderma, I feel I can cope with it better. I have learned to focus my energy in a positive manner, enjoying my hobbies and my children.

Some days are more difficult than others, but I go to the ISN's scleroderma message board and read the encouraging messages there, and that helps me. I am very grateful for each and every day.

David A. Wilcher
Diffuse Scleroderma
Ohio, USA

I am a lucky guy. But almost five years ago a few unlucky things started to happen.

Early in 1998, my hands became swollen, and I had a hard time gripping the handle of my coffee cup, so my doctor prescribed some water pills.

A few weeks later, my wife Toni and I traveled to Hawaii for our tenth wedding anniversary. We planned to do some hiking and backpacking. We had recently done a backpacking trip in Canyonlands National Park in Utah, and had a great time.

We drove our rental car to the trail head, somewhere on the big island. We parked and I grabbed my hiking boots, but my feet were so swollen that I couldn't get them on. Over next few days, my joints started to ache, and I could not get comfortable lying in bed. We had a good vacation, but we did not get to do all the things we had planned because I was not feeling up to it.

When I was back home, I went to the doctor when my fingers got infected. The doctor did a rheumatoid profile blood test, which slowed my antinuclear antibody (ANA) was very high at 1:2560! I was referred to a rheumatologist who told me he was pretty sure I had either lupus or mixed connective tissue disease.

Another month or two went by, and my rheumatologist noticed the skin on my forearms was getting tight and shiny. He sent me to see a doctor at the university, who did some more extensive blood work and found I had the SCL-70 antibody. She told me I had systemic scleroderma.

By this time my hands had started to curl up. I remember the G.I. Joe toys I played with when I was a child. The action figures were advertised as having "Kung fu grip!" because their hands were molded into a grasp to hold a pistol. So I started telling everyone I had *kung fu grip*.

My joints were aching, and I got very stiff. I had a hard time getting up and down and out of chairs. I could not even bend over to tie my shoes or put my socks on. I had difficulty swallowing and I choked easily.

The doctor at the university gave me some options, although none were proven to work. She told me about one drug which was very toxic. Another one was somewhat less toxic, and lastly, there was a controversial treatment using an antibiotic that only had some anecdotal success. At least it was not toxic, though.

At this point, I did not have any internal organ involvement other than my esophagus, so I opted for the antibiotic. I continued to work. I was a quality manager at a heat-treating company that hardened metals by heating them to high temperatures, and then cooling them. It was mostly a desk job, but I also ran a small lab. I had a difficult time reaching for supplies in overhead cabinets, and had to ask someone to get them for me. If I dropped a piece of paper on the floor it had to stay there until someone came by my office and I asked them for help.

A year went by and I got progressively worse. I changed my rheumatologist because the antibiotic was not working. Some days I would get home from work and I would be too tired to eat. I would get chills and could not get warm. I lost about forty-five pounds.

My lung doctor found I had only sixty percent of my lung capacity. My Raynaud's flared up, with my fingers turning purple, when things were stressful at work.

One day I was giving some important customers a tour of our workplace, when I started to feel very hot and had chest pain. After they left, I sat down for awhile and then I felt okay, but I decided to go to the doctor. They did a heart catheter, but no problems were found. My chest pain lessened over the next few weeks, and I'm convinced it was related to stress.

In January 2000, I quit working and applied for Social Security disability. The next month I went to the Cleveland Clinic on the advice of my family doctor, and they increased one of my medications.

Things have improved for me somewhat since then. I don't know if my improvement is due to the increased medication, or getting away from the stress of work, or just the natural course of the disease, as I have read that sometimes it stabilizes after four or five years. Regardless of the reason, I have less pain and my range of motion has improved. I still get tired easily, but now I can rest when I want.

I said, "I am a lucky guy," and here is why. I have a wife who loves me and takes care of me without complaint. She works to support us now that I no longer can.

My family has also been wonderful and supportive. They have helped me in many ways. I have a daughter who has become a wonderful young adult. She is twenty-one years old, and is fighting her own health battle. She just finished radiation treatment for Hodgkin's disease. She is going to beat it.

I have found that I can live with this disease, and I can also be happy. I have had to adjust my lifestyle, but it is a life I enjoy. There is great music, good books, wonderful movies, interesting people to talk to, and so many things to laugh about. I am a lucky guy!

Jennifer Weldon
Diffuse Scleroderma
California, USA

I am twenty-six years old. I was adventurous, energetic, and healthy prior to being stricken by two separate illnesses within the last two years.

I worked as a back office medical assistant nurse in an outpatient specialty department. On December 22, 1997, when I was twenty-four years old, I was rushed to the emergency room with severe flu-like symptoms. After I arrived at the hospital, all my vital signs dropped and my condition worsened.

After twelve hours, they concluded that an unknown virus was attacking my heart. I had every type of doctor working on me, but despite their efforts my body continued to shut down. My family was told I probably would die that night.

Fortunately, I made it to the next day, and they decided to transport me to the University of California, Los Angeles (UCLA) Medical Hospital. An aortic balloon pump was inserted into my right groin in hopes of keeping me alive while being transported. Upon my arrival at UCLA, I immediately underwent open-heart surgery for nine and a half hours, and I was placed on a biventricular mechanical heart machine.

I remained in a coma-like condition for two weeks. My lungs, liver and kidneys had all failed. I was on a ventilator and complete life support. I had five open-heart surgeries, and suffered severe nerve damage in my right leg. Eleven days later, my heart was taken off the machine and all my organs started functioning normally again. Six months after my release from UCLA, I returned to work part-time.

Then I started noticing pain and color changes in my fingers, and my hands seemed weaker, especially in the cold. I saw a rheumatologist and he diagnosed me with Raynaud's phenomenon.

Simple tasks became more difficult for me. In March, my arms became very itchy and started to tighten. Within two weeks my skin felt so tight that it was extremely painful. Soon I couldn't hold a toothbrush or tie my shoes. My hands and fingers felt cramped, and the skin was very sensitive. I called my cardiologists, since I thought this might be an aftermath of the heart failure, but they said it most likely had nothing to do with that.

I went back to my rheumatologist, and he said I might have an autoimmune deficiency disease, called systemic scleroderma. He referred me to Dr. Philip Clements at UCLA, who specializes in scleroderma. Unfortunately, the wait to see Dr. Clements was too long for me, considering the rapid pace of my illness, so instead I saw his associate, Dr. Ken Kalunian. After a few blood tests and a skin exam, he knew the diagnosis and wanted me to see Dr. Clements right away.

My parents, boyfriend and I met with both specialists. We discussed the possibility of a stem cell transplant, which is a new research protocol. The doctors were very concerned with the rapid progression of the tightening of my skin. They thought my organs would be affected if I waited too long, and that I had a good chance of dying within five years.

They urged me to be cautious and not make a hasty decision, due to the tremendous risk involved in having a stem cell transplant. Only one other person at UCLA had had the transplant for scleroderma, and he had died during the procedure.

Naturally I was scared and uncertain, and so was my family. But not having the transplant seemed more detrimental. There was no promise of curing the scleroderma, but there was hope that my pain might stop and that my skin might eventually soften.

We talked, prayed and cried, and in the end I decided to go ahead with the transplant. Then I met with Dr. Mary Territo, the oncologist who was in charge of my daily care. I had many blood tests, a bone marrow aspiration, lung function test, electrocardiogram (EKG), and even a cardiac stress test to determine if my heart could tolerate all the chemotherapy, radiation and ATG.

I was given injections to stimulate and quickly increase my stem cell count, and then I had my stem cells harvested. They inserted a catheter in my left groin to hook up the machine that sorted out my stem cells.

Once my count reached a certain level, I was admitted to UCLA hospital. They put a central line catheter in my chest, then I had two days of high-dose chemotherapy and two days of full-body radiation. I also had a few treatments of a medication called ATG.

This was done to make my blood counts reach zero. Then they gave me back my stem cells through the catheter. During this time while my blood counts were being restored, I was in the most danger of dying because my immune system was not fully functioning yet.

The third week, I developed a lot of fluid in my lungs along with an infection. They did a lavage of my lungs, which is a bronchoscopy, and gave me an intravenous diuretic. I had trouble breathing and I was scared that I was not going to make it.

Thankfully, after a few days my lungs started to clear and my counts were back up. On July 3, 1999, after a month in the hospital, I was able to go home.

I could not have made it through this without the constant love and support from my family and friends. My mom and boyfriend took turns staying with me overnight. The rest of my family, including my father, sister, brother, and sister in-law, comforted me during the long days.

I hope others with scleroderma will find the courage to have a stem cell transplant. If the doctors learn more about fighting and curing scleroderma this way, then my decision to have the transplant and to go on living will have been worth the fight.

These rapid-onset illnesses almost took my life twice, yet I have survived. I have learned how precious life is and how grateful I am to still be here. Now I am ready to live my life, and hopefully make the most of it.

Jo
Diffuse Scleroderma
Massachusetts, USA

Three months ago I was diagnosed with systemic sclerosis. I am a thirty-five year old woman with a four-year-old daughter. I have only been sick for ten months, so this is rapid onset.

Raynaud's came first. Within weeks I developed swelling and joint pain, and then a terrible pressure in my head. I have pain in the muscles of my eyes. It is not Sjögren's, it is inflammation in the eye muscles.

After about six months, I noticed that I could not make a fist. I did some research and then I knew what my diagnosis would be. By the time I was diagnosed, I had skin tightening up to my elbows and on my feet. Now I also have it on my stomach. My feet hurt so much that I have a hard time walking. I also have episodes of shortness of breath.

I am eagerly awaiting an appointment with Dr. Korn at Boston University Medical Center in a few weeks.

I cherish every day with my daughter and I only wish I had lived every day differently before I got sick. I also hope this is not hereditary, so that my daughter will never have to deal with this disease.

Lisa V.
Diffuse Scleroderma
Mississippi, USA

I am thirty-nine years old and I have had scleroderma for seven years. When I first got sick, I thought I was dying. My fingers started hurting really bad. I did not know what in the world was wrong with me. My doctor sent me to the emergency room, where an internal medicine specialist diagnosed me with Raynaud's. My doctor finally told me that I might die if I did not get to a rheumatologist soon.

I started out at a medical mall, until I got on disability, and then I found my own doctor. I have a great doctor who has been able to get my disease under control. Her name is Dr. Valee Harisdangkul. When I started seeing her, the scleroderma had already moved to my face. Since then it has moved back down to my elbows. My hands and arms are crippled.

In the last eight months I have felt better than I have since I have been sick. I am a survivor. I have a nineteen-year-old daughter, and a four-year-old grandson. They are worth fighting for!

For the first year I could not lay down or sleep. Now I am on medications for circulation, damaged nerve endings, skin ulcers, Raynaud's, and anxiety.

On my right hand, all my fingers are bent under, and my arms are contracted at the elbow. I type using one finger on my left hand.

My mother has been to every doctor appointment with me. We have traveled to Oxford, Tupelo, Tennessee, and back to Jackson, Mississippi, for treatment. She has stuck with me, even though I have been screaming in pain, day after day, and I have only been able to ride in a car only a short distance at a time before needing a break.

I love my mother. There is nothing better than having her at my side. She has probably heard and responded to my every cry. Thanks, Mom!

All my meanness as a teenager is paying off. I have strong will power, and my faith, without which I would have no hope.

Thank you for letting me share my feelings. I hope this will help somebody who is going through a similar thing.

◆❖◆

M. R. Sujatha
Diffuse Scleroderma
India

My name is Sujatha. I am thirty-six years old and hail from Bangalore in the southern state of Karnataka in India. I am ailing from diffuse systemic sclerosis. I thought that sharing my experience would be helpful to those who have the same illness.

In January 1992, my fingers turned blue occasionally. I consulted a reputed physician in Bangalore who said it was Raynaud's phenomenon. My cervical spine X ray showed slight constriction in blood supply originating from my right collarbone. I was told to consider surgery but I opted out. I was not put on any medication, but I was advised to avoid extremely cold conditions.

In July 1992, I observed a slight swelling in my neck. Routine thyroid tests like T3, T4 and TSH were done, but my thyroid was functioning normally.

We moved to Muscat near the end of 1992. I was not having any major problems as far as diffuse systemic sclerosis was concerned, but the Raynaud's still persisted. We moved to Dubai in 1994 and by mid-1995 I developed joint pain. I was advised to exercise regularly and was given a medication, which reduced the pain.

By mid-1996 my fingers were swollen, my face was tight, my nose was pinched, and my lips were drawn. Raynaud's was now affecting my hands and feet. This was when I was diagnosed with diffuse systemic sclerosis.

By August 1997, there was sporadic pitting of my fingertips owing to reduced blood circulation to the nerve endings. I was advised to regularly massage my hands and feet with olive oil and wear warm clothing, and I was started on more medication.

By October of 1998, we had moved to Kuwait, and there I was seen by doctors from the rheumatology department of a government hospital. I was advised to have regular blood tests and pulmonary function tests.

One of my medications gave me all sorts of side effects. I suffered from acute nausea throughout the day and could hardly eat anything. I started losing hair on my head and I went into premature menopause on account of the side effects.

Owing to premature menopause, I started getting regular hot flashes which continue to this day and is one of the most daunting and depressing of all my symptoms. In fact, at times I get the feeling that this has precedence over all other scleroderma-related problems.

We returned to India in November 2000. I hurt my left toe at a social gathering, and it itched accutely because of the local anesthetic which the doctor had prescribed. Nothing worked to cure my toe. I simply stopped most of my medications, and I stopped pouring water over my toe while having a bath. Simultaneously I started consulting a homeopath doctor. Ever since then, the toe, although not totally healed, is at least dry, but the pain still persists. Now, one of the toes in my right foot has started exhibiting similar symptoms!

The pitting or ulceration on my fingers is slightly worse now. I try to avoid chopping vegetables and have my maid do it. I regularly massage my hands and feet with lotion to keep them from feeling so dry.

I continue to see my rheumatologist and homeopath regularly. I hope and pray that I at least continue to stay the way I am and that I will be able to continue with my routine chores.

Mary J. Shaw
Diffuse Scleroderma
Louisiana, USA

I am fifty-seven years old and was diagnosed with diffuse scleroderma in 1998. In 1995, I was working as a supervisor at a local casino. I really enjoyed my job even though it entailed using chemicals.

In 1997, I began losing a lot of hair and weight, and I was always very tired. I blamed it on all the walking I had to do, although I had not lost weight before. My legs, ankles and feet had a very red rash that I could not get rid of, no matter what I tried. They felt like they were on fire and I often had to sit down as I felt I would fall from tiredness. My feet and hands also tingled with the burning and I was having awful pain.

I finally went to our family doctor because my husband was leaving for Venezuela in South America and I had to get a month's supply of his blood pressure medication for him. The doctor happened to notice my rash, and asked me about it. He ordered blood work and urine tests, put me on a diuretic for the swelling, and fussed at me for waiting so long.

I also have ulcerative colitis and it had given me a bad spell, so I was unable to go to work. The doctor told me he was looking for either a kidney or heart blockage and for diabetes, because it is common in my mother's family. He referred me to a highly regarded doctor.

This new doctor ordered more blood work and a scan of my legs. He did a biopsy in the deep muscle tissue of my right leg. My husband left for Venezuela the day before the biopsy. I was sent home after the surgery with pain medication and told to stay quiet. Each time I went to the doctor my pulse was very weak, and so was I. I asked when he thought I could go back to work and he said in ten to twelve days. That never happened. I had to walk on my tiptoes to get around, as the surgery site was very painful. By then my leg rash was a deeper red and had become scaly. My legs were tight and hurt badly.

When I had the stitches removed, the doctor put a gel on my legs and asked if I could feel it. I said no. He asked if my hands and feet were always so cold and I said yes. I asked if he had any idea what I had, but he still did not say anything about what was wrong with me. One day he said I had some calcinosis. He also thought he knew someone better than him who could get to the cause of my problem, and sent me to an internist.

The next two months I had more rounds of blood work, X rays and CAT scans. I was still losing weight and hair! I was in the office when he called the internist, and I heard him say, "I think I am sending you a patient who has scleroderma, but I am not sure. She has a lot of the symptoms."

This internist asked a lot of questions too. He asked about my hair, and how much weight I had lost. I told him I would bring him some of my lost hair on my next visit—and it turned out to be a gallon bag filled to the top! He increased my medication. He said the blood in my legs was terribly inflamed. I had no reflexes in my legs. The colitis was really acting up, but it will do that with stress, and I was certainly stressed. Yet I still had no answers.

The day finally came when he told me I had lupus. I knew what lupus was so I felt scared, but he assured me I could live with it. The internist made an appointment for me to see a rheumatologist.

When the time finally came for me to see the rheumatologist, I was a bundle of nerves. He told me I did not have lupus, that I had scleroderma. I did not even ask him what scleroderma was, since I was so relieved not to have lupus. But after he explained scleroderma to me, then I sure had reason to be scared. He put me on another medication. He told me to avoid scratching, to wear denim pants, and to stay as warm as possible. "In Louisiana?" I thought. Then he told me there was no cure for scleroderma, either.

My next appointment was with my old internist. When I told him what the rheumatologist had said, he laughed and said the other doctor, who he had referred me to in the first place, was right all along.

Since that time I have gone to the emergency room with a headache that I swore would kill me and with my chest hurting. It turned out I was having a migraine and severe acid reflux.

I also have fibromyalgia. I had an MRI for a herniated disc. I have a lot of degeneration in my left hip. I cannot wear my rings because my hands are swollen and hurt. My fingers and toes go into spasms and I have to push them back into place because they hurt and are crooked.

I had a barium swallow because I was coughing hard and felt like my throat was closing up. That was also due to spasms. I have peripheral neuropathy. I have Sjögren's, which causes dryness of my mouth, nose, lips and eyes. I no longer have any hair on my legs or underarms.

I have an inflamed tendon, which swells my foot up to the size of a loaf of bread and hurts a lot. I also have ear problems. The ever-present ulcerative colitis landed me in the hospital last year.

My family has been my lifeline. My husband took over so much, and it does not seem to bother him as much as it bothers me. He works in the Gulf of Mexico on an oil and gas production platform, so for a week at a time I am alone, but his family is nearby.

I walk with a cane and I have a wheelchair to use for long excursions. I am thankful for my husband and children who care and do so much for me.

I have learned to live with it by taking one day at a time. It is good to know that I am not alone in my struggle.

I try to keep a positive outlook on things and laugh about some of the things that happen. A little humor goes a long way. I have plenty of cats and dogs to keep me company, too! They in themselves are something to laugh at. These days, I would much rather laugh than cry.

Pamela W. Marshall
Diffuse Scleroderma
Texas, USA

I am forty-nine years old and have diffuse scleroderma with overlapping CREST. I was forty-four years old when I was diagnosed and heard those strange terms for the first time. My newlywed husband, of only two months, sat there looking at my doctor in complete bewilderment and all I could think was that it sounded pretty bad.

My doctor was ecstatic and ran out of the room to get some of his colleagues to take a look at his rare find, since none of them had ever seen scleroderma before. He tried to explain the illness to us, but we both were in too much shock to absorb it.

I remember thinking then that I had so much to be so happy about. I had a new grandchild, four great children, and a wonderful new husband, so why was I sick?

I went to a rheumatologist and after she had almost killed me with tests and medications for a year, she threw her hands up and said there was nothing else she could do, because I was getting worse and she had tried everything she could. She suggested that I go to Boston. Well, she might as well have said Japan, since I live in Texas!

Five years later, with the help of a few good doctors and many medications, I am still here, just not kicking! I have another grandchild, with another one due in April. I still have a wonderful, caring husband.

I have tackled this disease with jokes and laughter. It seems to help, especially with my husband and family, as I have to be strong for them. When I graduated from high school I was named "Miss Fun" and I was known as the "Carol Burnett" of the class.

Through all the trials and tribulations, I know that there must be a reason why I was picked to have this disease. When I get to heaven, that will be my first question. I am sure there will be a lot of us asking that!

◆ ❖ ◆

Sherrill Knaggs
Diffuse Scleroderma
New Zealand

I am fifty-five years old and live in New Zealand with my husband. We were commercial greenhouse tomato growers for twenty-two years.

In 1996 we took early retirement and moved to a small piece of land in the country bordering the sea. We had great plans for the future, but they all came to a grinding halt when I was diagnosed with diffuse systemic scleroderma.

About thirty-one years ago, when we had only been married a short time, I was diagnosed with Meniere's Disease, which left me deaf in my right ear. I have just recently learned that it is now classified as an autoimmune disease. I have also always had trouble with interstitial cystitis, which apparently falls into the same category.

I started getting a few symptoms of scleroderma about three years before I was diagnosed. My mother and grandfather both had severe Raynaud's in their hands and feet, so when I started having Raynaud's in my thumbs and index fingers during cold weather, I assumed it was hereditary.

I became fatigued, even though I previously had nearly unlimited energy. We had experienced about ten years of very stressful events in the family, so I thought that was the reason for my ongoing tiredness.

In June 1996, my Raynaud's worsened, with all my fingers going white, as well as my toes, earlobes, and the tip of my nose. Since we were having a rather cold winter in New Zealand, I still disregarded this.

Although I had not gained any weight, my wedding and engagement rings suddenly became so tight that I had to have them enlarged.

In August 1996, I mowed our lawn. The grass was long, the weather was hot, and it took me nearly two hours. Afterwards I was very tired, and my hands turned bright red and felt like they were on fire.

They remained so painful that I began wearing soft gloves for everything. Slowly they became stiffer, until I could not make a fist. By then it was difficult for me to even grasp the car steering wheel, so I put a sheepskin cover on it.

Eventually I went to a doctor. She did blood tests, and found my antinuclear antibodies (ANA) were positive at 1:640. My ANA later went to 1:1280, then 1:2560, and then back to 1:1280.

My feet became sore and I had pins and needles sensations in my hands, arms, legs and feet, chest, and face. I went to a neurologist, who did nerve testing with needles and electric currents, which was very painful, but the tests ruled out a neurological cause for my numbness and tingling.

Then I went to a rheumatologist, who said I had undifferentiated connective tissue disease (UCTD). I had never heard of that, and I did not want to take the medication he was recommending, so I asked to be sent to an immunologist.

The immunologist was puzzled, but wondered if I had scleroderma, and tried me on estrogen hormone. It caused me to swell up and feel terrible, so I stopped taking it.

I consulted a psychologist, since by this time I was wondering if any of this was in my mind, but they found no particular problem.

I still felt very ill and tired, so I started with another general practitioner, who thought I might have chronic fatigue syndrome (CFS). However, as I became worse he also began to wonder about scleroderma.

I saw another rheumatologist in May 1997. By this time I was having trouble walking, with sore feet and stiff knees. I had given up driving, and spent most of my time resting. My worst fears were realized when he diagnosed me with diffuse systemic scleroderma.

He gave me a variety of medications. After a week I felt much worse, so he doubled my dose of prednisone. That was years ago, and it put me in bed, and I am only starting to get out of bed a bit now! I weaned myself off the prednisone and did not go back to him.

My skin felt like plastic, stretched and tight, and it was hardening over most of my body. I had a dreadful itch along with severe sunburn-like pain, from head to toe. I had moisturizer applied at least twice a day, which afforded a little relief to the itch.

I could not straighten my arms because I had elbow contractures and a neck contracture. My hands resembled claws. My fingers were curling and my index fingers and left thumb were shortening. My knuckles and toes had little ulcers, and small bits of calcinosis.

My mouth became small, making it difficult to eat. I had no appetite, was continually nauseated, and I could not sleep.

I lost nearly seventy pounds, so I was down to ninety-five pounds, and I am five foot seven. My bones stuck out and I developed bedsores, so my husband made special foam pads for me to sit on and to rest my feet on.

My lungs had some fibrosis, and due to knee contractures I could no longer walk.

But the worst thing was the constant itch and pain. I was taking pain-killers around the clock, but without much effect. My doctor would not prescribe anything stronger, and because of the unrelenting pain, I really did not want to keep on living.

My husband was at his wit's end, and my eighty-year-old mother had shifted to live just along the road, so that she could help my husband look after me. Her husband, my father, had just died a few months before.

At last I found a compassionate doctor, who I still consult, who put me on stronger pain medication, and it was quite a relief, even though it did not completely quell the pain.

Our local hospice was a great help at this time. Those were dark years, and I did not want to see anyone except my husband and my mother, and definitely not a rheumatologist.

Somehow we struggled through, and the pain and itch started to lessen a little. In November 1999, my eyes became red and sore. I had not been out in a car for over two years, but I had to see an eye specialist.

I made it there with my husband's help, and was diagnosed with iritis, also called uveitis, another autoimmune disease. I was put on steroid drops and eye ointments, along with drops to keep my pupils dilated and to stop the swollen iris from sticking to the lens. This cleared up, but I had another attack, in one eye only, in September 2001.

In June 2000, my mother fell and broke her hip. She made a good recovery after her hip replacement, but we felt she should not have to look after me anymore. Since then I have had caregivers for six and a half hours every day, which is paid for in large part by Social Security. My husband looks after me the rest of the time.

In July 2000, my kidney function was declining, and my doctor persuaded me to see another rheumatologist, whom I still go to. My rheumatologist sent me for tests, and then to a renal specialist.

Due to scleroderma my kidneys had barely ten percent of function left, and I needed to go on kidney dialysis. After looking at the options, I chose peritoneal dialysis. In December 2000, I had the catheter placed for the dialysis and I began dialysis ten days later. As I am not able to set up the dialysis myself, my husband was trained on dialysis and handles all of it for me.

In March 2001, I received a cycler dialysis machine, which does the dialysis automatically at night, over the space of ten hours, so I am hooked up to it at night, and unhooked in the morning.

In April 2001, my hemoglobin dropped alarmingly low, and I was rushed to hospital for a blood transfusion of three units of blood. I had to stay in the hospital for many tests and a gastroscopy.

They didn't find the cause of my anemia, so I went home, only to have the same thing happen three weeks later. Altogether this happened five times.

Eventually they ruled out internal bleeding with another gastroscopy and a colonoscopy, and determined my anemia was due to a lack of erythropoietin. When kidneys fail, they often do not produce erythropoietin, which is the hormone that stimulates bone marrow to produce red blood cells.

Therefore I began getting erythropoietin hormone injections. About every six to nine months, depending on my ferritin level, I also have an iron infusion by IV. This replaces iron stores, which are used up in making hemoglobin. These two things have solved my anemia problem very nicely.

The gastroscopy showed some gastritis, so I was prescribed a medication to control stomach acid, which also relieved my heartburn. However the medication made my irritable bowel syndrome much worse, so eventually I stopped taking it.

In August 2001, my blood pressure shot up to 180/110. It is now well controlled with medication, and in fact it is almost too low.

In March 2002, an eye specialist told me that I have some degree of Sjögren's syndrome, which is another autoimmune disease. I need lubricating eye drops and ointments for this. I also have a rather dry mouth.

My improvement over the past year has been dramatic. When I last saw my rheumatologist he said my scleroderma seems to be "regressing."

He said they don't know what causes regression with scleroderma, they just know that it happens sometimes. He mentioned that the improvement usually starts at the head and works its way down, which is exactly what mine is doing.

My scalp used to be so tight that it was immovable. Now it moves normally, and my once straight hair has become very curly! This might be due to the collagen receding from my scalp, and twisting the hair follicles, giving me curly hair.

My dentist is amazed by the softening of my mouth. Tightness had ironed out all the wrinkles on my face, but now it is softening so much that I have wrinkles!

My arms are almost straight again. Although my hands are still difficult to use (I type with my thumbs and one index finger), my physiotherapist found that my hand measurements are getting better, and the muscles in my palms are returning.

I have gained twenty-five pounds. My lungs have improved, and my Raynaud's has lessened.

Although I still cannot walk, my legs are fifteen degrees straighter than a few months ago!

In June, my kidney function tests were better. My renal specialist said that if I continue to improve, and if I can get out of my wheelchair, they could then consider a kidney transplant for me.

I have very little pain and no itch now. Best of all, my brain is no longer in a grey fog!

Update – September 2002

I purchased an exercycle with a proper chair on it, as a regular seat would be too uncomfortable for me. I am pedaling a short while each day, as I do not want to overdo it and set myself back. I certainly could not have done this even a few months ago.

If I am going to walk again, I need to build the muscle tone in my legs, which the exercycle will do, and it will also stretch my legs some more.

I am having some trouble with high blood pressure. It began when they changed the brand of my erythropoietin, so I am off that for a month to see if it is the culprit. After only ten days my blood pressure is already dropping, so I may need to go back to the original brand.

I am steadily getting more wrinkles on my face as my skin continues to soften. Who would have thought that I would welcome this!

Much of this has happened since I volunteered to help on this Web site. I am sure that being motivated plays a large part in making me feel more positive, which in turn helps me heal.

I am also improving thanks to the constant support and help of my husband, my mother, my caregivers, and many friends who are praying for me; and, most of all, with the help of God.

Fellow sufferers of scleroderma, take heart, there is hope out there, and light at the end of the tunnel!

Becky H.
CREST Syndrome
Michigan, USA

My diagnosis was a long time in coming. I was diagnosed with CREST scleroderma in June 2002.

When I was nineteen and pregnant with my first child, I was diagnosed with rheumatoid arthritis. I was in a military hospital and they withdrew fluid from my joints, which had swollen to the size of baseballs. I was in tremendous pain. I never realized a person's bones could really hurt, even when they were sitting still.

They put me on aspirin every two hours around the clock. Then I found a book that said pregnant women should not take aspirin and I showed it to my doctor, so he put me on prednisone instead. After I gave birth, all my symptoms went away and I thought I was over it.

Four to five years later, I tested antinuclear antibody (ANA) positive for scleroderma in a pre-op blood test. I was going to nursing school, so I had all the scary information it to read. I saw a rheumatologist and he decided I just had a strange blood makeup because, as high as my titer was, I did not show any symptoms of the disease. Once again I thought I was home free.

Several years ago I started having problems with swallowing and had to have my esophagus dilated. The next year, at my son's football games my hands would become numb and painful and looked like they belonged on a corpse.

My primary physician has been taking care of me since I was a child and he basically dismissed my complaints about Raynaud's. Doctors do not like it when the patients make their own diagnosis, even if the patients are nurses.

Finally a new doctor came into the practice and took notice. He sent me to a rheumatologist again. I did not give it much thought, and I almost canceled the appointment because I had worked the whole night before, and was tired.

Like many nurses, I am a doctor's nightmare patient, because I never do everything they say and I treat symptoms myself whenever possible.

The doctor did a thorough exam and said, "You have scleroderma. This can be a very scary disease and not much is known about it. We need to get you on the right medications and prevent the symptoms from occurring. Most important though is that you check your blood pressure very regularly because hypertension is what usually kills people with scleroderma."

I had gone to this appointment by myself, and I freaked out. I called my husband and asked him to meet me at home right away. I asked the doctor if I should be scared and he just looked at me while I was crying, and he did not say a thing. That did not make me feel any better!

I started having panic attacks and began to search for everything I could on the disease. I dug into the Internet and every book I could find.

I took all the tests the doctor ordered. Suddenly I had doctor appointments almost every week, whereas before this I didn't even get a yearly physical on a regular basis.

I also had a problem with swallowing and they were telling me to take more pills, which I still never remember to do very well. My pulmonary function test showed minimal lung involvement, and they dilated my esophagus again.

After the busy time following my initial diagnosis, now I am just dealing with the changes as they occur and trying to keep depression at bay.

I have minimal involvement at this time, but gradually things keep getting a little worse. I have doubled up on my reflux medicine and I constantly battle the cold weather and the Raynaud's. But it could be worse.

As my pastor says, "What is the guarantee that any of us are going to be alive ten years from now? We have got to make the best of the good days we have when we have them."

I have two teenagers and an awesome husband of seventeen years. I am still a nurse, although I am trying to work less to decrease my stress.

◆ ❖ ◆

Carla Woodgate
CREST Syndrome
Minnesota, USA

All of these stories sound so different. I was hoping to read one of these stories where I could say, "Hey, that is exactly what is going on with me!" I see bits and pieces here and there, but there is nothing I can completely relate to. All the examples sound like the patient is quite ill and in extreme pain. I do not really have those problems anymore. I think I am quite healthy, even though I have been told otherwise.

I first recall having extreme pain in my hands and feet when I was a sophomore in high school. I had gone to Monte Cristo ski resort in northern Utah, which is a couple of hours from my home, and on my return trip, my hands and feet began to thaw. The pain was severe and I cried the whole way home.

I always had sores on my arms and legs like a rash. They were small bumps that resembled pimples.

When I was twenty-two (in 1979), I was in a car accident. I was badly injured, so everything that happened after that I blamed on the accident. I had pain and stiffness in my legs and back, and terrible headaches. I kept saying that you could not survive an accident like that and not expect some trouble.

I had two children, and then *five* miscarriages! I kept thinking it somehow had something to do with the car accident.

When I was thirty-one and expecting my third child, a doctor said I had the cardiolipin antibody and that it was probably causing the miscarriages. He put me on prednisone and heparin and I was able to go to term with the baby. Then I was tested regularly for this antibody. I later had a blood clot in my leg and was told that it too was a result of this antibody.

Then one morning, I woke up and was unable to raise my arms to brush my hair or hold my toothbrush. I went to see my general practitioner who sent me to a neurologist. He put me through some very painful tests and told me that I had multiple sclerosis (MS), totally ignoring a positive antinuclear antibody (ANA) test result.

For three years I went along thinking I had MS. Although I never had another episode like the one I woke up with, I did have pain and stiffness in my joints. I began having breathing problems and a simple cold would almost always result in pleurisy.

I saw a rheumatologist who began testing all over again, and took note of the ANA. There were few clear results, so I was told I had a lupus-like syndrome and fibromyalgia.

When I moved to Texas, I began to see another rheumatologist, who called it a mixture of connective tissue disorders, not mixed connective tissue disease (MCTD).

I went through a few years of trouble, mostly from the fibromyalgia. I also had some strange dizzy spells and disorientation that were determined by a neurologist to be complex migraines. She started me on medication for the seizures, and I never had another spell like that again.

In October 1999, I had surgery to remove a mucinous tumor from one ovary. It was a borderline malignancy, so my doctor did a complete hysterectomy, also removing my appendix, lymph nodes, and taking peritoneal biopsies, which were all benign. From that time on, my symptoms disappeared, aside from morning stiffness and sores on my arms, hands and torso.

I had been feeling very good for almost two years, but my doctor here in Florida kept telling me that I needed to see a rheumatologist, even though I was not having any trouble.

I went to see a respected doctor here and he went over my history and took a few more tests, which yielded some new results. Apparently, I have CREST syndrome, not lupus, not MS, not a mixture of whatever.

Do these things all overlap or mimic each other? I have a positive result on the SCL-70 test. What does that mean? The way my doctor talked, it was good news, compared to what they thought was wrong with me in the past. If I have CREST syndrome, will I develop scleroderma? Is that what the SCL-70 test implies?

Why would my doctor suggest that CREST is better than lupus? It sure does not look that way to me! I have been viewing some web sites, reading histories, and seeing pictures, and I am not too thrilled about this. Frankly, some of these stories scare the devil out of me.

I am so bewildered. I keep getting my diagnosis altered and I am just ready to pull my hair out. Why has this been so hard to pin down?

◆ ❖ ◆

Chelle
CREST Syndrome
Tennessee, USA

When I was sixteen, I was rather heavy, and I just about quit eating to lose weight. I went from two hundred down to one hundred and fourteen pounds in just a little over six weeks. I thought I looked good, but my family felt differently. I don't know if that was the reason I got this disease, but my doctor said it did not help.

I became very tired, and I thought it was due to my lack of nutrition. I also lost some flexibility in my muscles and joints.

My family kept pleading with me to go to the doctor, and finally I did, about a year or so later. They said the itchy line of dry skin across my belly was just a fungus, and that I needed to exercise more and eat better.

A few months later, I could not hold down a job. I was dizzy and tired and sick, and too run down to make it through the day. Finally I was sent to a doctor who knew what I had and confirmed it with a blood test! You have to specifically be tested for scleroderma.

When I learned about all the things that happen to people with scleroderma, I gave up and waited to die. Then one day I decided to get up and get moving. I started taking a bath and dressing myself again. I have been in remission for about eleven years now. My scleroderma is just external. My hands and my face are mildly affected.

My CREST symptoms include tiny red dots that appear on my hands, as well as red blotches on my face and nose. I have Raynaud's, which causes my hands turn blue to purple, and I am sensitive to cold. I also have calcium deposits on my hands, and arthritis.

I am doing fine now. I have learned to live with the few symptoms I have and I remember that there are others worse than me.

I started eating again, and I went back to work. It is possible to have a life with scleroderma. However long we have, we can just make the best of it.

◆ ❖ ◆

Dawn Sinclair
CREST Syndrome
Scotland

After two major operations at the end of 1995, I had severe chest pain, very much like angina. I was very unwell throughout 1996. I began to have severe sweats, aching muscles, and very crackly joints. I also developed eye and skin problems. These things have continued for seven years now.

I have had many medical tests. Initially, when the tests came back negative, my symptoms were put down to anxiety so I visited two psychologists over a period of four years. The psychologists always felt that my problem was physical, but my doctors stuck firmly to the belief that it was psychological.

I was trying to take care of my two children on just child support income. Since I did not have a diagnosis, I could not get the help I needed, and at times I was in utter despair. After five years, I asked my general practitioner for a diagnosis, but he refused to answer my questions, so I went to the health council and they wrote letters on my behalf. To cut a long story short, I was struck off my doctor's list.

Within a few months, my new doctor diagnosed cervical spondylosis and found that I was having internal bleeding. I have lost the core stability muscles in my lower back due to pain.

Recently I developed lumps on my elbows, knees and ankles. I have Raynaud's, I get very breathless, and I do not have the stamina I used to have. I had tests done this week to see if I have CREST syndrome, since I also have Raynaud's.

I feel hurt that no one has cared enough to help me, and I feel sorry that my two children's lives have been affected by it. My fear is that more damage has been done because my illness has been allowed to go on for so long without proper medical treatment.

If you suspect that you have this illness, pursue it as vigorously as you can. Do not allow the doctors to dismiss you. If they will not listen to you, trust your intuition, and change your doctor.

◆ ❖ ◆

Dianne M. Rutherford
CREST Syndrome
Canada

I was diagnosed with CREST and pulmonary fibrosis twelve years ago. I worked as a graphic and commercial artist until three years ago, and was the art director of a medium-sized lithographic company. Like many others, I was misdiagnosed for over twenty years.

I was first told I had arthritis and then rheumatoid arthritis. Lupus was also diagnosed, and I was given treatments for them all. Nothing helped and I only got worse. My general practitioner had no idea what was wrong with me. I used to feel upset when I left his office, as I knew he did not believe what I was telling him.

Twelve years ago, I went into a crisis. I was running a very high fever and my kidneys were shutting down. I was taken to the local hospital where the emergency room doctor told me outright that he had no idea what was wrong with me or how to treat me and that I should see my general practitioner about a reference to a specialist and go home and rest.

My old general practitioner had retired and, thankfully, my new general practitioner was more aggressive. He sent me to one of the large downtown hospitals and to the best specialist in this city.

The specialist ran many tests; including X rays and blood and urine tests. After seven hours, he called my older sister and me in and told us that I had scleroderma with CREST and pulmonary fibrosis. We had never heard of scleroderma before. This diagnosis opened a whole new world to both my family and me.

For nine years had regular three-month follow-up appointments with him and also regular pulmonary tests, CT scans, and blood and urine tests. I tried enough medications to choke a horse but nothing other than prednisone seemed to help.

While I knew the scleroderma was progressing and I could feel it, others did not notice. I looked too healthy to be sick and I refused to give in. I had a demanding job, lived on my own, traveled and also had a cottage.

I nursed my mother through her heart problems until her death, and nursed my older brother through colon cancer for two years until his death. I also looked after my mother's older sister in a nursing home. Then, on December 28, 1999, I went into heart failure.

Suddenly, my disease hit me in the face. I was sent to see another specialist at another hospital in the city, who told me I was a perfect candidate for a double-lung transplant. After a year and a half of testing and many hospital stays, I was informed they could not do the transplant, but to, "Stay in touch. We may have a new drug for you to test out for us."

I went back to my original specialist and my general practitioner. I was discouraged and angry. My general practitioner was disgusted at the way I was treated and could not believe that they offered no follow-up.

This June I went into another crisis. I had a massive gastrointestinal infection. My liver and kidneys were a mess and I was having mild heart attacks from the heart failure. Again, they rushed me to the hospital.

This time I had no pulse and my blood pressure was forty-five over zero. The emergency room doctors worked to get me back and I spent another week in the hospital. Thank goodness my local hospital had improved since my last visit twelve years earlier. The doctors were wonderful. However, they got no help from the downtown hospital, since they still will not release my medical records.

Now I am much worse. I get very short of breath, the edema is a battle and the water pills are not working. I have more reflux and am on an medicine to help control it. I am also on many other medications. I cannot tolerate beta-blockers for my heart problems, but I always carry nitroglycerin with me. Last week I had another ultrasound and they found cysts in my kidneys, which is yet another hurdle.

My younger sister has moved in with me to help. She is very good, but has trouble understanding my "off" days. I still drive my car when she is not using it, and since quitting work I was asked to take over as president of the Board of Directors of our high-rise condominium. There are great people on the board and they help me a lot. It also gives me an outside interest and stops me from dwelling on my problems. I still love to cook and force myself to try to eat a healthy diet with no added salt and lots of fresh fruit and veggies.

I guess I look a bit sicker than before, since people can tell if I am having a good day or not and they ask how I am *really* feeling.

I try to keep a good sense of humor. My friends tell me I am a bit warped when I tell them the stories of what I am going through. The doctors have given me six months, but what do they know? Twelve years ago they told me I would never see fifty and I have beaten that by three years.

My specialist says my attitude just blows him away. As I tell him, everyone has problems. Some of us just have bigger ones to deal with.

I sold the cottage, which broke my heart, but I just could not look after it and it is not fair to have to ask others to do it for me.

I miss not being able to come and go as I please, and now I sometimes my sister has to push me in my wheelchair as I just cannot walk very far any more. However, my little Shih Tzu dog thinks the wheelchair is a great mode of travel, as she sits on my knees.

I am just glad that this crummy disease is getting more exposure. Now other people have at least heard of it, even if they do not know what it is all about.

Elaine Pero
CREST Syndrome
Canada

I was diagnosed with scleroderma in the winter of 1986, in Calgary, Alberta, Canada. I started having stomach problems when I was twenty years old. My fingers would turn waxy white and feel so cold that at first I thought I had gotten frostbite.

Over the years I developed lumps on my knees, elbows, wrists and fingers. In 1985, while on vacation in Saginaw Michigan, I awoke at four in the morning, feeling fine. When I woke again at eight, my left arm was warm to the touch and so swollen that I couldn't bend it. Every bump in the road on the trip home was agony for me.

I was given the wrong antibiotic at first, and I was sure I was going to lose that arm, since it had swollen to twice its normal size. Luckily it cleared up, but it took almost two months.

That started a long era of testing. I was sent for tests in Hamilton, Ontario, but it wasn't until we moved to Calgary, after a week in the hospital and numerous calcium infections, that I was diagnosed with the CREST syndrome of scleroderma.

I had two operations to remove calcium deposits in my hands so I could keep on working, because I love my job as a chef. I had operations on both of my knees, as well. Sometimes it hurts me to walk, get in the car, or even turn over in bed because of the calcium build-up in my hips.

I can't take many medications, as I am prone to horrible side effects, so I have opted to suffer with pain rather than feel sick all the time. I am still working and I hope they will do another operation on my right hand so that I can continue to work. My left hand has now started to develop ulcers as well.

Between gastroesophageal reflux and all the other complications of this disease, it gets frustrating some days, but I figure it could be a lot worse.

I am glad I can still work, and still do the gardening that I love. It hurts for me to bend over, so what used to be simple is now a chore, but the results still make it all worthwhile.

I am fortunate that my husband is very understanding. Over the years he has always been there for me, through good and bad times. My mother-in-law is also a jewel. I wouldn't have made it without their support.

I know it will get worse, but I try to focus on the happy times and the good things, rather than on myself or my disease. I really wish that they would find a cure for this.

Jan M. Landis
CREST Syndrome
Oregon, USA

In 1977, I woke up on a summer morning with my fingertips purple and hurting. The only way I could describe the pain was that it felt as if I had grabbed a hot pan.

My family doctor thought it was Raynaud's, and he referred me to the research center of our local university hospital. I spent four years as a guinea pig doing their ice tests, which consisted of measuring the temperature of my fingers, then dipping my hands in ice water for thirty seconds, and then measuring the temperature again until they returned to normal temperature, which rarely happened within their two-hour testing period.

My life was hectic during those years. I was raising three boys including his, mine, and ours, and trying to hold a job when I could.

Eventually, I began to see a rheumatologist because of lesions on my fingers, which caused excruciating pain. I applied for Social Security disability in 1986, but was told that I should still be able to find a job I could do. I let it slide since we were preparing to move across country.

In our new hometown I was shuffled from one doctor to another because we had no medical insurance, so I was again seeing doctors in a teaching university, and that is where I was finally diagnosed with CREST.

I went to work again, but after six weeks I was in such pain that I could no longer work, and it took nine months for my hands to finally heal. I applied for disability again, and received it.

After five years in the Midwest, we moved back to the West coast where the weather was more moderate and better for my health.

I started having breathing problems three years ago. I would become short of breath if I did much walking. I chalked it up to being a smoker, but when I mentioned it to my doctor, he ran some tests.

My lung function had diminished and my X rays showed fibrosis. My doctor gave me two options. My first option was to do nothing, and the second was to start chemotherapy, which might have a twenty percent chance of doing any good. Since it was my only hope, I began chemotherapy in January of 2000. I see my doctor every three months for a treatment and check-up.

I am feeling better now than I have in years. I haven't had any flares since I started the treatments. My breathing hasn't improved, but it hasn't deteriorated either, which to me is just as good!

I want to let everyone who is suffering through these terrible things know that we should never give up hope.

We should set goals, even short ones. My first goal was to see my youngest son graduate from high school, which he did in 1997! Now I have another goal, which is to live to see my twenty-fifth wedding anniversary in June of 2004. I will be there!

Jeff Armstrong
CREST Syndrome
Canada

Two weeks ago I was diagnosed with scleroderma, after seven years of severe Raynaud's. My rheumatologist said I have CREST, or limited scleroderma, and to see him again in two months. I originally went to see him for an infected ulcer on the end of one finger which I thought was a complication from the Raynaud's.

Since I had never heard of scleroderma, I didn't ask any questions when he told me about it, and instead I came home and looked it up on the Internet. I certainly found a lot of information, and did not really like what I found.

Now I am having a hard time thinking about anything else. After reading about the symptoms, I discovered a few things that I have had for years that may be related to this, like heartburn, problems swallowing, and red dots on my hands.

I am a thirty-seven years old, with a wife and two very young children. I rarely ever missed a day from work on the local auto assembly line. My wife and I have long-term goals and plan things out well in advance. We try to do all the responsible things like retirement and education planning.

Now my world has been rocked. I have missed eight weeks of work and I do not know if I will be able to continue doing the type of work I have done since I was eighteen.

I feel like I have run into a wall at this point, and I am looking for a door that will let me continue with my life as I had planned it. I have made an appointment with another rheumatologist who specializes in scleroderma, but will have to wait another ten weeks for that.

In the meantime, I am on a roller coaster of fear, depression and confusion. What a ride.

◆ ❖ ◆

Jill Carpenter
CREST and Sjogren's Syndrome
England

I am fifty, and I have had severe Raynaud's since early childhood. The doctors told my mother it looked like Raynaud's but it could not be since children do not get Raynaud's, so it was probably a sign of good health!

I suffered dismally but learned to accept my lot. I was bullied at school because kids assumed I did not wash properly as my skin was a dingy color. I in the loo (restroom) during physical education class. I sat in the loo and snuck back in when the lesson was over.

By the age of fourteen I had leg ulcers and was in the hospital for some time for tests. They said it was just a reaction to puberty and that I would grow out of it.

I learned to skip school and became a rebel. To put no finer point on things, in the era of "peace and love" I found my own "cure." It was very risky and illegal, but it made me feel better than I had for years.

I grew out of my rebellion and put all that behind me, and then I felt exhausted, tired and depressed once again. I became bluer than ever all over, not just my hands and feet. I felt this was my own fault so I put up with it.

I had trouble working. I would need to take time off, as I was too tired to put one foot in front of the other. I did temporary work instead as the money was very good and I could choose your own hours, within reason.

I was diagnosed with depression and given electroconvulsive therapy (ECT), and tranquilizers in vast quantities. I learned in later years that this was an experimental approach that was finally abandoned—thank goodness! I was told it would clear my mind.

The experimental ECT treatment left me with another legacy, which is hard to handle. Follow up research has found that it caused the same things in others, too. Anyway I digress.

In 1977, I had an accident and fractured my pelvis and was taken to the hospital. When it was X rayed they found some calcium deposits.

A renal specialist thought my color indicated Brights disease, but he referred me to a cardiovascular doctor who referred me to a "friend" who had an interest in Raynaud's.

The upshot was that I was in danger of losing my lower left leg and toes. My right foot and all my fingers were infected and ulcerated. I had learned to live with it because after all, it was just due to depression!

I was rushed to see a professor in a London hospital who performed a bilateral sympathectomy. I was sent home with pneumonia two months later.

I did not get any better, so I went back to the hospital to be treated for the pneumonia and also had a bilateral cervical sympathectomy. This time I was a lot better, and I basked in the feeling that at last I could start living. The pain and things I was left with were a small worry now. I could even cope with the exhaustion!

My left hand was still bad after a few months, so they redid the sympathectomy on that side. The operation did not go well and I ended up with pleural pneumonia, and it took me a long time to recuperate.

Six months later I suffered from peripheral neuropathy and I became paralyzed in the extremities. I was in the hospital for some time, but they eventually decided it was hysterical paralysis since I had a history of depression. Isn't hindsight a wonderful thing? Peripheral neuropathy is now recognized as part of scleroderma.

Eventually I was mobile again, although I still did not feel well. Once again, I learned to live with it. I adapted to my own way of getting by.

In 1980, I had to have a medical exam. I saw my medical records said I had Raynaud's, but what was scleroderma? I had never heard of it. I assumed it must be part of the Raynaud's, so I never asked. By this time I was doctor-phobic and I was sure everything was all in my mind and that it was my own fault.

I steered clear of all doctors for many years. I went to see my dentist because I was suffering badly with mouth problems. She was horrified and sent me to the dental school at Guys Hospital in London. They realized I had no saliva and then looked for tears; none there either. I was diagnosed with Sjogren's. Still, no link was made to the Raynaud's. I ended up losing all my teeth.

I had the most appalling obstetric history with several complicated pregnancies and deliveries and many miscarriages. My obstetrician wanted me to see a rheumatologist but by this time I declined and discharged myself. I gave up trying to have babies! That way, I did not have to go to the hospital.

In 1988, I was rushed to the hospital for an emergency hysterectomy as I was hemorrhaging. Once again they asked me to see a rheumatologist. This time I agreed. The rheumatologist was wonderful. He explained to me what scleroderma was, and said he was certain I have CREST.

Then he dropped a bombshell. I waited for him to say he would make it all go away, but instead he wanted me in for tests. I panicked. I could not face being in or visiting a hospital anymore, so I discharged myself from his care.

I decided that as I have lived with it this long I will simply get on with it again! Since then I have had general practitioner care only. She is well informed and knowledgeable and acts as an intermediary between me and the hospital.

Kathy Baker
CREST Syndrome
Texas, USA

I live in Houston, Texas. I was diagnosed with CREST scleroderma on June 18, 1997. Before that, I had problems for six years with red, white, and blue fingers that were painful.

I had stomach ulcers and esophageal reflux spasms that sometimes caused me to wind up in the emergency room for a gastrointestinal cocktail and a shot. When I ate half of a sandwich it felt like I had eaten three.

Food would become stuck between my esophagus and stomach, so I would stick my finger down my throat to regurgitate to relieve the pressure. That way I wouldn't wake up in the middle of the night choking on all the stomach acid.

My gastrointestinal doctor did an endoscopy and found eight stomach ulcers and seven esophageal ulcers. He treated me with medication and a bland diet.

This worked for about a year until the symptoms worsened. He then ordered an esophageal motility test. They ran a long rubber tube down my nose through my throat and into my stomach. I swallowed sips of water as they pulled the tube up a little at a time and took pictures on the monitor.

When the test came back my doctor said, "Kathy, either this test is wrong and we need to do it over, or you might have scleroderma."

I said, "Sclero *what?*" They ran the antinuclear antibody (ANA) blood test. On June 18, 1997, my doctor's nurse called me at work and said, "Kathy, your test came back positive for scleroderma. You need to see a rheumatologist, but we can't get you in to see him for two weeks. And hopefully it is in remission."

I asked her, "What is scleroderma?"

She stated, "We don't know much about it, so you will have to see the other doctor."

So I went Internet surfing! I found a lot of information, but not knowing which form of the disease I had was frustrating and scary.

I walked into the rheumatologist's office wearing shorts. My legs were covered in purple splotches and my fingers were blue. His first words were, "You definitely have Raynaud's."

I said, "Cool. Now tell me what that means."

My final diagnosis was systemic scleroderma CREST. He taught me about scleroderma and how to take better care of myself. He prescribed several medications for my symptoms.

I had some side effects so my medications were changed. I refused to take other medications, and the symptoms returned. It seemed like a revolving door, but I learned to deal with the disease and now it is a normal part of my life.

I entered a research study here in Houston. I have one of the best rheumatologists in the city, and a good gastrointestinal doctor. My gynecologist says autoimmune disease threw me into early menopause.

Many of my teeth have been pulled due to absorbtion of the jawbone from scleroderma, and more of them are loosening. Eventually they will all probably need to be pulled.

I have poor intestinal motility so I have to take prescription laxatives every day. In 2001, I had surgery as a result of the slowed motility.

The skin on my fingers has become thicker and shinier, and my fingers are harder to bend. The calcinosis sores on my fingers became painful.

This year one of the calcinosis sores became so infected that I was hospitalized. They discussed possible amputation, and did surgery. Luckily they only cut out the infected section down to the bone in my thumb.

I was in the hospital for four days, plus I had home care health nurses for a week to change the packing and bandages, and another week of occupational therapy after that. The wound looks good now and is finally healing.

If I sit too long my knees hurt, and I look like Grandma Moses getting up off the couch, but once I am up and running I am good to go. I have chronic fatigue and sometimes it just comes in waves. When I have eaten too late in the day, I sleep sitting up to prevent choking at night.

I get toe ulcers that often take months to heal. Sometimes I wonder if amputation will eventually be the only remaining option. I also have digital pitting which is making the tips of my fingers deteriorate.

Thankfully I live in Houston where the weather is hot ten months of the year. I love the heat! My coworkers have a hard time being in my office because I always keep the space heater on so my fingers will not ache and go through the "patriotic" color changes of Raynaud's.

I have a great support system with my husband, family and friends.I don't feel sorry for myself because I believe I was given this disease for a reason. I may not know the reason yet, but I'm sure I will know it someday. Maybe it is to share my story so others don't feel so alone in this fight, and to help educate the public on this rare and little-known disease.

For me, scleroderma has been a roller coaster ride emotionally and physically, but I know it could be worse. I am fortunate to still be able to work full-time, even though I have setbacks periodically, and the pleasure of visiting the hospital for a few days. At least that gets me out of cooking dinner and cleaning house!

Kristen Scala
CREST Syndrome
Maryland, USA

I am still rather new to all of this, but I feel like I have been living with CREST forever.

Two years ago, my general practitioner sent me to a rheumatologist because I had elevated antinuclear antibodies (ANA). I was just told I might have osteoarthritis (at thirty-five?) and sent home.

My pain continued and the swelling increased. My chiropractor knew something was up, as he diagnosed my Raynaud's.

A year and a half later, my new rheumatologist diagnosed me with CREST. I didn't know whether to cry over the diagnosis, or feel relieved that I wasn't crazy.

Then I began to read up on CREST. Now sometimes I worry about how long I will live with this, and who would take care of my children if something happened to me. I really want to live long enough to see them graduate from high school.

I have been switched from one medicine to another since I was diagnosed, but nothing seems to stop the acid reflux. My swelling has continued, so other medications have been added for that.

I know it could be worse. I read other people's stories and I am thankful, and scared. I just need to be grateful for the time I do have. Sometimes it is hard. But ask me how I'm doing in a year, as I will still be here!

Marie
CREST Syndrome
Florida, USA

I am forty-six years old, and I have been married for twenty-eight years to a very special man, and we have three daughters.

About ten years ago I had a nodule on my thyroid which was biopsied and Hashimoto's thyroiditis was diagnosed. I was put on thyroid medication and the nodule mostly disappeared.

About eight years ago my fingers began turning numb and white when I was shopping in the grocery store freezer section and when it was cold outside.

I also began having trouble swallowing pills sometimes. My migraines worsened and I was put on a medication in hopes of stopping them, but they did not go away.

My doctor sent me to an endocrinologist who said my swallowing problem—which had escalated to choking on liquids—might be early scleroderma. I didn't know what scleroderma was, so I started researching it while I was waiting for my blood test results.

It turned out I had a positive antinuclear antibody (ANA) in the centromere pattern, which is associated with CREST syndrome, so I was sent to a rheumatologist. He did a nailbed capillary test and exam, and confirmed that I had CREST syndrome.

I was taken off of the migraine medication since it might have been worsening my swallowing problem. I was pretty good for several years, but the headaches were horrendous and would last for days, and the Raynaud's became worse. Sometimes there is a lot of hesitation before I can swallow, which makes me fear choking.

I had a flare of Hashimoto's which was much worse and the fatigue was relentless. The nodule reappeared and became painful to touch, so they increased my thyroid medication. They wanted me to take prednisone, but I was too scared of it, so I settled for a nonsteroidal anti-inflammatory (NSAID). It took five weeks for improvement, so I might have compromised my recovery by not taking the prednisone.

Chronic fatigue is my worst problem now. It seems to grab on and not let go. I work full time as dental office manager, which thankfully is mostly sedentary work, however, when I come home and have to face dinner, dishes, and laundry, the fatigue puts me in a horrible mood. Usually I am too tired to even think about doing any of it.

Since I have started taking antioxidant vitamins, most of my symptoms have improved. Maybe it is just a temporary thing, however my rheumatologist and my primary doctor both think that I look pretty good for having had scleroderma this long.

My nail bed capillary test improved so much that my doctor ordered a new ANA test, but it indicated my disease has escalated and become more active, even though I haven't noticed any changes.

McKenzie A. Graye
CREST Syndrome
Montana, USA

I was standing in the kitchen of my home in Seattle, Washington, and talking on the phone with my daughter, when I felt numbness crept down both my legs. I said, "I can't feel my legs!" and sat down on the floor. My daughter called 911, and I was taken to the nearest emergency room.

The doctor took one look at me and started asking questions about the red "butterfly" pattern on my face.

"Why are you concerned about my face, when my legs are the problem?" I asked.

"I'm going to do a blood test," was his answer. A few minutes later I was told I had antinuclear antibodies (ANA) in my blood and that I probably had lupus. They referred me to a rheumatologist.

From the rheumatologist I learned I have scleroderma with CREST. I had never heard of scleroderma. I knew that I had dry eyes and I had been diagnosed several years earlier with Raynaud's, but I had no idea they were related to an autoimmune disease. The doctor gave me several pamphlets along with a prescription for artificial tears, and I was sent on my way.

I believe in meeting an enemy head on, even if the enemy is my own body, so I began researching scleroderma. Scleroderma is a rare disease and information on it was scarce in 1993.

At that time my worst problem was fatigue. I had no energy and my joints hurt all the time. My eyes felt like they had sand in them, due to the Sjögren's.

My life consisted of going to work, coming home, and going to bed. I was always exhausted. Housework did not get done. I had no social life, no hobbies, and no interests. It took such an effort to just exist. If a flu circulated through the department where I worked, I would not only be sure to catch it, but I would also be slower to recover than anyone else.

Raynaud's was also a problem. My fingers would turn transparent white, all the way up to my palms. I would lose feeling in my fingers. Wearing gloves did not help. Stress, caffeine and rainy weather seemed to be the triggers. I would run warm water over my hands until the blood came back into my fingers, which hurt a lot. I learned biofeedback to bring the blood back into my fingers in a less painful way.

Degenerative disc disease, which is inherent in everyone, can be exacerbated by Sjögren's. The fluid in two of my discs dried up and they bulged, one of them pinching my sciatic nerve. I was unable to work and after a long hard battle with the long-term disability insurance company, I was able to quit work. Disability pay was half my regular income, so I began looking for an inexpensive place to move, someplace quiet with little stress, because stress speeds up the progression of scleroderma. I moved to a little town in Montana called Hungry Horse.

I was extremely lucky to find a wonderful family doctor. She treated me for depression, and tried several antirheumatic medications, but unfortunately they did not help me. She told me that good nutrition was important and recommended multivitamins and vitamin B. The vitamins have helped my energy problem and even though I am still tired most of the time, I have moments when I am able to enjoy a hobby.

The dryness in my eyes worsened to the point where I had to use eye drops constantly. Reading was out of the question and I found myself sleeping more, just because it hurt to keep my eyes open. I mentioned this to my opthalmologist and he suggested plugs in the lower tear ducts.

The plugs helped for a year, and then it worsened again, so I had both the upper and lower tear ducts in both eyes cauterized. Now I have just enough tears to keep my eyes moist without spilling down my face. I sure hope a cure for it is found soon, because there is no next step if my tears dry up more.

Swallowing is difficult for me, so I mostly eat soft, moist foods. I have heartburn. All the discs in my back have degenerated, so I am in constant pain and cannot sit, stand or walk for over half an hour. Some nights I hurt so much that I cannot sleep.

A month ago I noticed that the inside and top of my right foot was constantly numb. My doctor referred me to a neurosurgeon. After studying an MRI of my back, he told me there is no nerve impingement and the numbness is probably due to the scleroderma. There is also the possibility of multiple sclerosis (MS), which is another autoimmune disease, so he ordered an MRI of my brain. There are cases of scleroderma plus CREST, where another autoimmune disease is present. I am hoping this is not the case with me.

Now I would like to focus on the positive side of having scleroderma. Yes, there is always a positive side. Once I got over the shock of learning that I have an autoimmune disease, I had two options. I could sit around and wait to die while whining about the symptoms, or I could live each day to the fullest.

Every day is a gift and I look for the good in each one. Watching a mama bird bring her little ones to my bird feeder, enjoying the way the sunlight plays on the leaves of a tree, getting hugs from my kitten, these things are precious to me.

I am closer to family and friends and have learned to be nonjudgmental and to love them as they are, for their friendship is priceless.

So many of us get so wrapped up in our own bubble gum that we forget to stop and wonder at the beauty and love that surrounds us. Having scleroderma has made me appreciate the little things and my life is richer for it.

Everyone on this earth has something difficult to overcome. These things will make us stronger and bring out the best in us, if we let them.

Renae Boswell
CREST and Sjögren's Syndrome
Iowa, USA

I was diagnosed with scleroderma about four years ago at the University of Iowa Hospitals in Iowa City, Iowa. I was referred there by my doctor after undergoing an endoscopy for problems with swallowing and keeping down food as well as severe acid reflux.

After my second endoscopy, the rheumatologist asked me questions about the past several years, including how my hands and feet reacted to cold, and if I had noticed any stiffness and pain in my hands, joints and muscles. I had always attributed these things to getting older, and I thought my blue fingers were signs of carpal tunnel from my years of secretarial work.

The rheumatologist asked if he could perform a little test on my hands with cold water, and I agreed. He had six resident doctors watch as he dipped my hand into a bowl of ice water. After about fifteen seconds I had to remove my hand. My fingers were white and painful. Then they turned blue, then red.

The doctors were excited and examined my fingertips under a magnifier and also mentioned a narrowing of the fingertips and tightness of the skin on my fingers. I left the hospital being told that I most likely had scleroderma. They wanted me back the following week for blood work and a stomach emptying study.

I drove the ninety miles home by myself worrying and fighting back tears. I had no idea what scleroderma was. The next week, I learned more, and I have since received most of my information from Web sites and from questions I asked my doctors.

I have suffered many complications with the Sjögren's. I had tear ducts in both eyes cauterized due to extreme dryness. I had oral surgery for ulcers on my tongue. I have a stone in my parotid gland that causes severe bouts of pain and swelling. My dental problems have been constant and severe. I am lucky to have a dentist who has researched Sjögren's in order to treat my condition.

I have severe dry skin and problems with rashes. I take a medication to help alleviate some of the dryness. I continually need liquids to help me swallow food and keep my mouth moist.

I even need fluids at night because the dryness causes my tongue to stick to the top of my mouth, which disrupts my sleep. I use special toothpaste for dry mouth, and do daily fluoride treatments.

My Raynaud's is mostly apparent in colder weather and when air conditioning is too cold. I take medication for it, and I use special care to protect my fingers and toes from the cold.

My esophageal problems are quite severe. I take medication for acid reflux. I must continually drink water to push down my food, as one-third of my esophagus does not function. I do not eat after five or six o'clock at night because of food coming back up when I go to bed. I have an ongoing problem with constipation,. so stool softeners are a daily necessity.

My hands, arms, joints, and muscles in general are painful. I am treated with an antirheumatic medication two times daily. Being tired is a constant problem; it seems I run out of steam often.

I have spots on both legs, around my shin bones. They are red and circular, indented, and hard on the surface. My rheumatologist said they are localized scleroderma. I was given an ointment to ease the dryness, but sometimes the spots are very painful and it feels as if the pain goes into the bone.

Recently my blood pressure has been very high, and medication has brought it under control. This has been a concern as my blood pressure has been on the low side my entire life, and I worry about the possibility of pulmonary hypertension (PH).

I do not know if heredity is a factor in scleroderma or not. I have a very dear younger female cousin who has CREST scleroderma. She was recently diagnosed with stage four pulmonary hypertension. I pray for her every day. She is a mother of two teenage girls who need her so much. She was diagnosed about twelve years ago.

Basically, I consider myself to be very lucky. I still work every day, and I rarely miss work, except for doctor appointments. I am grateful for good caring doctors, and for all the good days, as well.

◆❖◆

Theresa
CREST Syndrome
Maryland, USA

I am fifty years old and I was diagnosed with CREST in September of 1996. I had no idea what CREST was, so my doctor told me to go home and look it up on the Internet, which I did.

My symptoms started with my hands and feet. They turn white with cold and bright red with heat, and it is very painful. I also began having shortness of breath and acid reflux. Now I use inhalers twice a day, and take medication for the reflux.

The skin around my fingers is often dry. It cracks open and takes awhile to heal. I also have painful stiff joints in my fingers, hips, arms and knees.

I am a cake decorator and I am not ready to give up working, even though my job causes a great deal of my pain due to the constant squeezing of icing bags and going in and out of the refrigerators.

When I get home from work, I usually go straight to bed because of the pain. I have been told to stop this kind of work, but it is all I know. I did manage to stay at home for six weeks one time, but I could not handle thinking about my situation, so I went back to work.

I do not know what my outlook is. I only know that I am constantly in pain. Being busy is the only way out for me, so I also teach Bible study for children at my church.

It is my faith in God that keeps me going when the medicine doesn't work or when my doctors say there are no silver bullets for curing this illness. My faith gives me the strength to get up on cold rainy days when I am in pain. It pushes and pulls me through each and every day to encourage others who are worse off than me, and gives me rest for my soul and spirit.

◆ ❖ ◆

CHAPTER 4

In Remembrance

She taught me what relentless meant
by fighting for every moment of life.
—Cheryl Delane Robinson

Cheryl Delane Robinson
Mother, Systemic Scleroderma
Texas, USA

This is what I shared at my mother's memorial service.

Some of the last words my mother said to me were to tell me how special I was to her and how much she loved me. She and my father adopted me when she was twenty-nine years old. Her doctor had told her that carrying another child would be too much of a risk to her health so she chose to adopt because, as she said, she wanted a daughter.

In the last weeks of her life I drove from Austin to Houston every few days and spent the night at the hospital once a week with her. There was someone from our church or family with her twenty-four hours a day. She was in so much pain during this time that all I could do was brace myself for a night of staring helplessly at her, as she could not find a moment's peace. My mother, who always had the answer for any problem, was the source of my security. She taught me what relentless meant by fighting for every moment of life.

Could this even be happening? As I stood staring, I finally admitted to myself that she was not going to win this battle. At least not win it the way I needed her to. I needed her to look at me and reassure me that she would always be there for me and that this was just another hospital stay and this was just like the triple bypass, the hip replacement, the several surgeries ensuing the hip replacement, the hand amputation and all the other procedures she had endured, and that she would be coming home.

I wanted to be able to hear her laugh and talk to our family cat that she adored. I wanted her to ask me to sit on her bed in the morning while she drank the coffee I brought her. I wanted to feel her put her arms around me. I swore that I would do anything, anything at all if she did not die. I would quit my job and move home, be a better daughter, go to church more, live the way she had always wanted me to. I would do anything if she would just stay alive.

I felt so scared. What would life be like without her? How could I ever be happy? Why had I ever fought with her? What were the fights even about? I could not remember.

Why hadn't I said all the things I wanted to say now, before? Does she know how much I love her? Did she realize that when I was twelve and said I hated her that I didn't ever mean it? Why had I pulled away from her so much?

Around three o'clock in the morning when all her pain medication finally gave her a reprieve, she looked over and asked me to sit next to her so that she could see me. She told me, "The day that the lawyer brought you to us, there were so many people at our home waiting for you." I had heard this story a million times, but this time I opened myself up and listened. I knew that it would be the last time I might ever hear her tell it. I had often wondered why she told it to me over and over, but I finally understood that she wanted me to remember how important a day it had been for her.

She went on to tell me how it had all been part of God's plan. I was meant to be her daughter and she was meant to be my mother. She expressed gratitude to my biological mother for giving me to her.

I finally broke down and cried out, "You are my mother. The only one that I have ever wanted and I do not know what I will do without you!" She began to cry and said, "You still have your father and your brother."

"It will not be the same," I said.

"I know," she smiled, "I know." She asked me to promise her that I would be happy. She said that one day there would be a man in my life who would love me as I deserved, but that no one would ever love me as much as she did.

She was not afraid to die. She knew that God would take care of her. I thought to myself how amazing my mother was because I was mad at God. So mad that at the time I did not want to even think about Him. What was He doing? This is something that I still struggle with. My father, brother, her sister and I were able to see her before her last amputation. I was crying and she simply smiled and said, "No tears."

We have come together today out of love and respect for the most important woman in my family's life, my mother. The pride I feel for being her daughter extends beyond my ability to measure and at the same time, the loss I feel is sometimes unbearable.

The comfort that sustains our family comes from knowing that she is no longer suffering as she did for so long and also from the memories we have been able to share and the prayers that have been said on her and our behalf. Although my fear of this very day has been with me for far too long,

I have to fall back on what she has told me so many times before: "Stand up, be strong," she would say, "and do what you know in your heart is right."

What my heart tells me is right today, is very simple. Ensure that she is remembered for the amazing force that she was her whole life, not what her illness tried to make her. I watched my mother—with her engaging smile even when her pain was immense—greet people who came to visit or stay with her in the hospital.

She would tell the women how pretty they looked, or just how good it was to see them. She would tell the nurses she appreciated their care. I watched her reach up and touch one young nurse on the face and tell her how beautiful she was. She always made people around her feel happy.

My mother always told me how valuable good friends were and that if you were lucky enough you would have a few on whom you could always depend on. Please look around to see how many of you are here today. I ask you, how lucky was my mother? Feel blessed that you have been touched by one of the kindest souls this world has ever known. You have touched her life as well.

If she were here, she would hug each one of you and thank you for loving and caring for her and her family. Remember the good times of friendship and games, weddings and birthday parties. When you see her favorite things like elephants, giraffes, lighthouses and roses, think of her and feel joy that you knew her and that she is in a better place, free from pain.

Remember she was an artist, she loved to travel, and Barbara Streisand was her favorite singer. Remember she was always a Dallas Cowboys fan, even when they could not win a game. Remember her wonderful laugh.

Please remind her grandchildren how in love she was with them. She always said that you could never tell a child you loved them too often.

My mother passed away with the same grace with which she lived her whole life. We can continue on with the lessons she taught us. We can love each other, help each other and always be patient with each other. Brighten someone's day and never take for granted a day that we are healthy.

May I say one more time how proud my brother and I are to call her our mother. What a bittersweet day.

◆❖◆

June
Husband, Pulmonary Fibrosis
England

My husband, Eddy, died on April 7, 2002, after over a year of suffering, which was very severe in the latter months. We had both been married before and the tenth of July would have been our seventh wedding anniversary.

Eddy seemed to literally suffocate to death from pulmonary fibrosis, which in the early stages was diagnosed as mild asthma, and fluid on the lungs, and heart failure.

Eddy had a history of heart problems including several heart attacks, the last of which was in May 1997. He did not make much progress and was frequently hospitalized with low blood pressure and chest pain. We now know that the low blood pressure was worsened by some of his medications.

He was given many chest X rays and spent about three weeks of last year in the hospital, but it wasn't until he had the CT scan that pulmonary fibrosis was finally diagnosed. By then, his lungs were very small and his heart was enlarged.

Over the past year, Eddy went downhill very fast. It got to the stage where he was almost permanently reliant on home oxygen, and after several chest infections, he was taken into hospital two weeks before he died.

Eddy was seventy-eight. He had not smoked for about forty years, and he had never smoked heavily. He only smoked a pipe and an occasional cigar (but never cigarettes) while he was in the Royal Air Force and for a few years after being discharged.

It was suggested that his illness could have been the result of working in the laboratory of the local paper mill for over thirty years and inhaling paper fibers, but, of course, it could not be proved, since we didn't know of anyone else in a similar situation.

I watched Eddy change from an active, vigorous, jovial man who loved cycling and walking and lived a healthy lifestyle—apart from his great love of fish and chips and toffees, which I succeeded in modifying to some extent—to a man who became a shadow of his former self, insecure and agitated because he couldn't do the things he had always done so easily.

During his last few months he was virtually bedridden and completely dependent upon oxygen. One large cylinder would last him approximately twenty-four hours.

He was very brave and tried to maintain his sense of humor, but once when I told him how brave he was, he admitted that he was terrified. He kept saying, "I will get better," and, "When I'm better we'll do this or that." He wanted so much to go back to visit places that he had known as a boy. He even wanted to take me to Paris!

All I wanted was for a miracle to happen and have Eddy back to his old self, but it was not to be.

One of the most awful symptoms of the illness, which Eddy also found very distressing, was the terrible rasping noise that accompanied his every breath.

His last outing was on our weekly "Dial-a-Ride" Bus, which took us from home to our local supermarket and back again. During his last weeks at home, he was able to go only accompanied by a portable cylinder of oxygen. The courage he showed when walking out to the gate to get onto the bus was unbelievable. He then had to get from the supermarket to the bus and from the bus along our garden path to the front door.

On his last trip, much to Eddy's 'shame', as he put it, we had to borrow a wheelchair. He just collapsed into the front door and onto the sofa, fighting for every breath.

By then he was unable to get in and out of the bathtub, and the fact that he had to rely on me for a daily bed-bath (as he was always fastidious about personal hygiene) depressed and humiliated him to such an extent that on two occasions he declared that he wished he were dead. But then he said immediately, "Sorry, God, I didn't mean that."

My deepest regret is that I was not with him when he died. The hospital rang to say he was deteriorating. I called a taxi, but all the traffic lights were red and I arrived fifteen minutes too late. I find it very difficult to come to terms with the fact that I did not say goodbye to him and tell him I loved him one last time.

I know that I am not the only person to have lost a loved one to this terrible disease, but life is so empty without him. Thankfully, I have two lovely daughters, a very kind son-in-law, and three beautiful grandchildren, the eldest of whom, incidentally, has cystic fibrosis.

◆ ❖ ◆

Noreen
Daughter, Fibrosing Alveolitis
England

I would love to tell you about our daughter Alana Kate, who was born December 9, 1983, and died February 18, 1985. She was so brave and beautiful!

We have a son, Luke, who was born at twenty-eight weeks. He is now twenty-two years old and fine. We decided to try for another baby, but unfortunately I ended up having six miscarriages.

After the sixth miscarriage, we decided to have one more try, and I found I was having Alana. I had to have a stitch put in at thirteen weeks. I was on bed rest for the rest of my pregnancy, and I had to have a cesarean section.

When Alana was born she started having breathing problems and had to be put on a ventilator. At twelve weeks, she had a lung biopsy. This told us that she had fibrosing alveolitis. We were totally devastated when we knew she was going to die.

Alana gave us the most precious fourteen months of our life. She always had a smile for everyone, and because of Alana we now look after profoundly handicapped children.

Salina Saenz
Grandmother, Systemic Scleroderma
California, USA

My grandma died about two years ago from scleroderma. I am not sure when she was diagnosed, but I was in the sixth grade when we found out she was sick.

Since I was a child then, no one really explained it to me. All I knew was that she could not digest her food properly. She was fine for a few years. Then when I was a freshman in high school, she got sick again. This is when I started noticing that she was very sick.

My mom and I would go over and take care of her every Sunday. At first she could not keep food in her system and she lost a lot of weight. She was in the hospital a lot.

They wanted to keep her on tubal feeding so she could get food in her system, so they kept a tube in her chest for a while. Next her joints stopped working and her skin was hardening. During this whole time she was still losing weight. Just going over from week to week and seeing her slowly disappear hurt everyone.

The medical bills were too much for my grandpa. Grandma had to have special kinds of spoons and forks to eat with. She used eight different medications to help her go to the bathroom and to do normal everyday things. She also had a new kind of bed.

All of this cost money. They asked my grandma's daughters to help pay for some of her needs, which caused family arguments. My grandma was getting so sick that the doctor said to keep her in the hospital or get her a home care nurse. So they got her a home care nurse.

But still every Sunday, my mom and I would go help her. We had to help her do everything and she would get mad because all she wanted to do was be able to eat by herself and be able to play with my little cousin, but she could not.

All the medicine she took made her see things that were not there. I remember one time when we were going to lay her down for bed and she started pulling away saying, "The ants, the ants." She was scared to lie down because she thought there were ants on the bed. Sometimes she would start talking about a baby and asking, "Who is going to pick up the baby?"

When it got near the end, some of my aunts would not go see her because they did not want to see her like that. It was to the point where my mom would ask me, "Are you sure you want to see her?"

And I would go. I had to go to be there with her. I loved her. My grandma would always tell me that when she goes, she wants me and everyone else to remember how she was when she was not sick, how she was when she would laugh and go out to the movies with us.

She died in September. It was one of those days I will never forget. I was going to go to school, but I had this feeling like I had to see her. As my mom and dad and I were just about to leave to visit her, the phone rang. I was in the bathroom. All I heard was my mom crying and saying, "She is gone, she is gone." And with that I knew she was dead.

I rode with my aunt on the way over there. We talked about her and mostly cried. We got there and seeing her lying on her bed not breathing made me cry even more.

I was hoping she would start breathing again, but she never did. My other aunt had been there when she died. She had died in her sleep like she had always wanted to, with no pain or hurt. She liked to sleep because she said she could not feel any pain when she slept.

She is now safe in heaven, where she is at peace.

Shirley Sutton
Husband, Systemic Scleroderma
Canada

My husband John had scleroderma, and he passed away on November 8, 2001. He had scleroderma since 1985, for sixteen years. He also had lupus.

He was a hunter and golfer. He enjoyed riding his Honda Goldwing motorcyle and his all terrain vehicle (ATV) right up until the end. There are many stories I could tell, but the most important was that he never let scleroderma get him down.

To all those with scleroderma, please live life to the fullest, and may all of you be blessed.

PART 2

Juvenile and Localized Scleroderma

CHAPTER 5

Juvenile Scleroderma

*It amazes me how quickly one
can adapt to change, as long
as it is for the better.*

—Mary-Charlotte

Medical Overview of Juvenile Scleroderma (JSD)
by Dr. L. Nandini Moorthy

Dr. Moorthy is Assistant Professor of Pediatric Rheumatology at UMDNJ/Robert Wood Johnson Medical School in New Brunswick, New Jersey. As a pediatric rheumatologist, she is interested in taking care of children and improving their quality of life.

Juvenile Scleroderma

Scleroderma is an expansive term comprising of an assortment of rare chronic autoimmune diseases of unknown cause. These diseases can be broadly classified under the two main categories of local and systemic forms.

The localized form, usually mild, is only occasionally associated with other organ involvement. Examples include morphea, linear scleroderma, linear scleroderma en coup de sabre, Parry Romberg Syndrome, and other overlap syndromes.

The systemic form includes systemic sclerosis with diffuse scleroderma and systemic sclerosis with limited scleroderma. Limited scleroderma was once called CREST syndrome (**C**alcinosis, **R**aynaud's phenomenon, **E**sophageal dysmotility, **S**clerodactyly, and **T**elangiectasia).

Systemic sclerosis often causes severe organ involvement. It is crucial to distinguish between these diverse forms of scleroderma as they all have different clinical features, treatments and prognoses.

Localized Scleroderma

Morphea is the most commonly prevalent of the localized "scleroder-matous" diseases. Usually these children have irregular patches of thickened skin, most commonly on the trunk but sometimes on the limbs as well.

In linear scleroderma, the pattern of involvement is more in a line over one arm or leg and usually only one side of the body is involved. The lesion can start as an oval or round patch in morphea and linear band-like patches in linear scleroderma.

The lesions can be of different sizes, and are usually waxy, hardened, and pinkish-purple in color with a surrounding reddish halo. Some of these lesions may expand over a period of months to years.

Over several years, the lesion heals with a whitish scar and causes either hyper- or hypo-pigmentation depending upon the skin color of the child. The depth and extent of involvement varies, either being limited to the skin alone or extending more deeply even to the bone and leading to significant deformity and disability.

Routine laboratory test results, including complete blood count, urine analysis and chemistries, are generally within normal limits. Sometimes, the erythrocyte sedimentation rate (ESR) and immunoglobulin G level may be elevated. Rheumatoid factor and antinuclear antibodies (ANA) may be positive. Antibodies to denatured DNA and interleukin-2 receptor may used to follow disease activity over time.

Applying topical emollients should suffice for very small lesions that have stopped enlarging and do not hamper physical function. However, if the lesions are spreading, treatment options such as methotrexate, etanercept, Rocaltrol, Singulair and hydroxychloroquine may be considered. These lesions may be cosmetically undesirable, impede physical function, and cause contractures, particularly if they cross over the joints.

In a growing child, linear scleroderma of the leg can result in leg-length discrepancy. The prognosis of children is usually excellent unless there is significant involvement of muscle and bone or if the lesions are large and cross multiple joints, in which case surgical correction may be necessary.

The affected skin should be cared for and prevented from getting injured because optimum healing may not take place. Usually children with localized scleroderma do not have any internal organ involvement and do not develop systemic sclerosis. However, these children require thorough evaluation and continued monitoring by a pediatric rheumatologist.

En coup de sabre lesion is a type of linear scleroderma distinguished by a scar extending from the scalp to the forehead. Initially it appears as a thickened area of skin and over time, the scar softens.

Parry Romberg syndrome constitutes progressive facial hemiatrophy and can be associated with lesions in the brain and these children may have learning disabilities. In this syndrome the entire half of the face is affected as compared to the en coup de sabre where only the forehead is affected. Usually these lesions appear at one to two years of age. Affected children require routine neurological and ophthalmological monitoring. If cosmetic improvements are necessary, children may require surgical intervention by experienced plastic surgeons.

Children with localized forms of scleroderma require constant support and guidance in connection with their interactions with friends and families, as well as in responding to any questions they may have regarding their disease and apparently different appearance.

Raynaud's Phenomenon

Before talking about the systemic form of scleroderma, it is important to discuss Raynaud's phenomenon. In 1862, Maurice Raynaud described a three-stage series of color changes of the fingers and toes occurring in response to environmental cold and emotional stress. Although not all persons with Raynaud's phenomenon have all three color changes, the classic sequence involves blanching or whitening followed by a dusky blue-purple phase and in some individuals a third phase of exaggerated redness as blood flow returns to the fingers. Associated symptoms include pain, numbness and burning.

Blood flow to the fingers and toes is ordinarily around forty to fifty fold of that required for nutrition and oxygen supply. In cold environments, our body tends to limit blood flow to the extremities of our body, while in warm environments blood flow is increased to the hands and feet. In this way, the body can carefully regulate the core body temperature for optimum organ function. Due to the reduction of blood flow in the extremities of individuals with Raynaud's phenomenon, they are unusually sensitive to even minor temperature changes and have difficulties with simple tasks like holding iced drinks or reaching into a freezer.

Raynaud recognized that the phenomenon could occur as an isolated clinical problem in persons otherwise healthy but that it was also a sign of systemic illness. Modern physicians view Raynaud's phenomenon in much the same way.

An estimated ten percent or more of the healthy population, including both men and women, experience Raynaud's phenomenon. In these persons said to have primary Raynaud's phenomenon, the blood vessels are structurally normal but seem to have a heightened response to environmental stress. In this "haystack" of a very common complaint lies the "needle" of secondary Raynaud's phenomenon.

Secondary Raynaud's occurs when the blood vessels have been damaged or narrowed. In this instance, normal levels of blood vessel closure in response to cold superimposed on the narrowing lead to blockage of blood flow to the fingertips.

Prominent amongst the causes of secondary Raynaud's phenomenon is the systemic form of scleroderma. Raynaud's phenomenon is the most common presenting complaint in scleroderma and ultimately develops in nearly all patients, adult and children.

Individual episodes of Raynaud's phenomenon do not worsen the disease. Treatment of Raynaud's phenomenon is driven by the following goals: 1) to maximize patient function 2) to reduce symptoms and 3) to prevent digital ulcers.

Around one-third of individuals with scleroderma develop a fingertip ulcer at least once a year. Inadequate blood flow is the primary basis for the formation of these ulcers, although poor health of local skin tissues also contributes to the same. A patient with scleroderma who develops fingertip ulcers is well advised to treat their circulation and skin integrity with great care, in much the way a diabetic manages foot care.

Commonly used medications are vasodilators that increase the diameter of the blood vessel. Since the quality of life is improved with medications, these are considered beneficial.

However, not all patients with Raynaud's phenomenon need medication. Keeping the central body warm with layered clothing, wearing hats to minimize heat loss through the scalp, careful planning of daily activities to avoid cold exposure are three simple recommendations to cope. In some ways, Raynaud's severity is under the control of the patient. For example, if a medication is working, that individual may decide to risk more cold weather activities and thus risk more Raynaud's attacks.

Systemic Forms of Scleroderma

Systemic sclerosis with either limited or diffuse scleroderma is a chronic multisystemic disease that implies both skin thickening and organ involvement, most commonly of the lungs.

Children often present with shortness of breath. The most common presenting feature is Raynaud's phenomenon followed by tightness of skin and stiffness of the underlying joint. Skin tightening may be accompanied by sores over fingertips, rash over knuckles and nail-fold capillary abnormalities. Affected children may gradually develop difficulty swallowing and chest pain. Since the lungs, heart, kidneys, and the gastrointestinal system can be involved, these children need comprehensive evaluation and monitoring by a pediatric rheumatologist.

Usually, the routine laboratory test results are within normal limits, although muscle enzymes may be elevated. Certain antibodies such as antinuclear antibody, anti-DNA antibody, rheumatoid factor and anti-SCL-70 antibody may be positive.

Because of increased risk of lung involvement, these children may require monitoring with pulmonary function tests and high resolution CT scans. Heart problems may arise in parallel with or independently of lung involvement.

Children may need daily antacids and motility agents for gastro-esophageal reflux and to help the food pass through. Children who develop renal hypertension may require antihypertensives. In rare cases, they may develop scleroderma renal crisis, which is usually controlled by ACE inhibitors, a class of antihypertensive agents.

Limited scleroderma or CREST syndrome is a type of systemic sclerosis which comprises of calcinosis (calcium deposits under skin), Raynaud's phenomenon, esophageal dysmotility, sclerodactyly (tight skin over fingers) and telangiectasias (abnormal blood vessels that are visible reddish blotches). Children with this syndrome often have anti-centromere antibodies.

The goal treatment of the systemic form is to prevent internal organ damage. Depending upon the severity and extent of organ involvement, treatment options include hydroxychloroquine, methotrexate, cyclosporine, cyclophosphamide, and anti-tumor necrosis factor alpha agents. Over time, the skin thickening improves, but for children with internal organ involvement requiring aggressive therapy, prognosis may be more guarded.

Disorders such as mixed connective tissue disease (MCTD) and dermatomyositis may share several characteristics with systemic scleroderma and require appropriate management and monitoring. Eosinophilic fasciitis is a rare entity where the affected child complains of swelling, pain and redness of the extremity.

Further Reading

1) James T. Cassidy and Ross E. Petty. "The Systemic Sclerodermas and Related Disorders" p505-533; Audrey M. Nelson. "Localized Sclerodermas" p535-543; James T. Cassidy and Ross E. Petty. "Overlap Syndromes" p544-552. *Textbook of Pediatric Rheumatology, Fourth Edition,* Cassidy and Petty, Saunders Publishers 2001.

2) Thomas J. A. Lehman, MD., *It's Not Just Growing Pains—A Guide to Childhood Muscle, Bone, and Joint Pain, Rheumatic Diseases and the Latest Treatments,* Oxford University Press 2004.

◆❖◆

Ariel
Linear Morphea
Washington, D.C., USA

I am fourteen years old and about two years ago was diagnosed with linear morphea on my right arm. Luckily it only affects my skin so I can continue with my hobbies of dancing and playing the piano.

I started using a prescription cream about six months after the disease was diagnosed, but unfortunately there weren't any noticeable improvements.

My doctor then suggested PUVA light therapy. However, in the area in which I was living at the time, there was no UVA-1 light, so the doctors created a protocol for just regular UVA light. The light caused second-degree burns on my arm through a mistake in carrying out the treatment.

Now, six months later, I have tried to use the prescription cream again, but my skin still cannot tolerate it. Because of that, we are thinking about starting PUVA light therapy again, and I would like to know if anyone has tried this and has experienced any improvements.

Bianca
Morphea
Canada

My family started noticing dark silver spots on the side of my thumb when I was around four years old. I am now seventeen and there are countless scars on my body.

When I lived back home in Nepal, my parents always took me to doctors since the first appearance of morphea. They just thought it was something that would go away in a couple of months or years. Having heard that, they never seemed to pay much attention to it. But as I got older, the scars did not disappear, but started getting bigger.

It also caused problems with the way I walked when it started disfiguring my legs and my arms. As a result, my left leg and my right hand are a little smaller than my other leg and hand. Besides that, I also recently got new scars around my waist and breasts.

My parents took me to Japan and other countries to get good treatment. But no one seemed to have any answers for the behavior of those scars.

When I finally came to Canada, I was diagnosed with morphea. As I was fourteen at that time, it did not bother me much. I was already used to the discoloration of my skin.

I started becoming more aware of it later on that year. Now I feel really bad about it. I am seventeen and reading all these stories about death from scleroderma and it really scares me.*

I know there is no cure for it. I am still under observation and have to go to the hospital every six months. This disease not only scarred me physically, but mentally too.

Nevertheless, I have started to accept my body. I feel like I am not the only one who does not understand this disease when I read through all these stories.

A lot of these stories have touched me deeply. Whether I get the right treatment or not, I will not let this disease ruin my life.

Editor's Note: Morphea is a form of localized scleroderma. It is only occasionally associated with other organ involvement.

Chiara
Morphea
Italy

This story was translated from Italian to English by Kevin Howell. He is a Clinical Scientist for Professor Black at the Royal Free Hospital in London. The Italian version of this story is in Chapter 10.

My name is Chiara, I am nineteen years old and I have had localized scleroderma, morphea, for fourteen years. In all this time I seem to have done nothing more than "jump" from one hospital to another!

I was at a hospital where they "tortured" me with cortisone injections. Finally, after almost four years of treatments, my last hope arrived in the form of the "De Marchi" Hospital in Milan. Here the doctors managed to stop the disease, which is a great victory after so many years of suffering!

Debbie Wilson
Daughter, En Coup de Sabre
Canada

When my daughter was about five, we noticed the first of many lesions on her body. Although we went to our pediatrician and a dermatologist, it was not until she was eight years old that I noticed atrophy in her face. An en coup de sabre developed, and she was finally diagnosed with linear scleroderma. After every possible test was run, systemic scleroderma was ruled out, thank goodness!

Because my daughter's face was being affected so severely—with atrophy, hair loss, and partial loss of her eyebrow—we began a treatment program. For two years she had intravenous steroids for three months, followed by a year of injected methotrexate, and then a year of oral methotrexate.

She has been off the medication for two years now. The drugs did help. However, last month our worst fears were realized when two new lesions developed.

We are awaiting our next appointment, but in the meantime I was wondering if anyone else has experienced a similar situation. I have just read some of these stories. It really does help to know we are not alone. It is scary to think of going through this all over again.

◆ ❖ ◆

Ewa
Son Albert, Linear
Poland

This story was translated from Polish into English by Dr. Roy Smith and Dr. Magdalena Dziadzio. See Chapter 11 for the Polish version.

My experience of scleroderma started four and a half years ago in November 1997. At that time our son Albert was born, our long awaited and beloved child. In the beginning, that is to say in his first month, our life was a fairy tale, unimaginable happiness and good fortune that we had this beautiful and strong little boy, 4000 g birth weight and 57 cm long at birth. According to the APGAR scale he had 8 points at birth, but, so what? A bluish leg and a problem with his testicles, it was nothing and in fact, his testicles came back to normal in a week. His little leg did not. One month after his birth little Albert was referred to hospital with aspiration pneumonia: he was always coughing up milk when he was feeding, but he was growing normally and put on 2 kg in a month. And that is the end and the beginning.

Albert's father's concern that one leg was thinner than the other was dismissed by Albert's doctor as being a part of Albert's nature, and the fact that the skin of one of his legs was marbled was again "inventing a disease in a child." After a week in the hospital, Albert's father and I were exhausted and questioning what was happening and why the doctors behaved as they did. We lived like that for a year and nothing particular happened.

At three months Albert was sitting, after nine months he was walking and by one year he was an active walker, but he did not speak and was often ill. Besides that everything was going very well, with the exception of our trip to the children's hospital where many tests were performed to discover why one of his legs was dry, gray and rather marbled, a little bit deformed and thin, whilst the other was pink, soft and plump as a baby's should be.

When Albert was fifteen months old we noticed that he was behaving in a strange way and when I spoke to his doctor, he said it might be epilepsy, but not to worry. I could not stop thinking about this opinion and I took my son to be seen privately by a pediatric neurologist in Olsztyn. There, after having listened to me, the doctor sent him immediately for an EEG. It turned out that my instinct was right and that Albert really suffers from epilepsy. It was fortunate that I observed his symptoms early; as he has been taking drugs since and everything is now okay.

In the meantime, on his sick leg, a 1.5 x 2 cm lesion appeared; it looked strange surrounded by a red "frame," thick, rough, and itchy. I saw a dermatologist who prescribed a cream. At the beginning there was an improvement because the lesion was not red anymore; but unfortunately, when the cream was applied it was causing him pain and burning. Furthermore, Albert started to wake screaming to say that his entire leg hurt him! That seemed strange, so the dermatologist was changing the creams, prescribing different lotions and bath oils with no effect, while the lesion was growing and growing and the pain was getting stronger and stronger.

In the meantime, Asia, Albert's sister, was born, but despite it Albert was not weaned until he was four years old. One day Asia got a generalized rash.

My husband and I decided to see a dermatologist in Olsztyn. And then it happened! After we had entered the office, it turned out that Asia's rash was due to something I had eaten, but when I asked the doctor to give an opinion on Albert's problem, without much thought she called a rheumatologist for consultation. At the end I sat and cried and the doctor was writing a referral for Warsaw as Albert was diagnosed with scleroderma.

I did not know what this disease was but the doctor said, "If we manage to organize everything quickly, nothing bad will happen to him, but this is an incurable disease, and in some cases is fatal." This sentence only caused me not to be able to control my tears, and I already I hated this scleroderma.

We traveled to Warsaw where one doctor started to yell at us saying that it is too late, and that it was very bad that Albert had been vaccinated and so on. Later on in a hospital room when I asked, "What does scleroderma mean?" I heard a sentence that was the beginning of the end: "I know some people who like Albert have scleroderma and despite it have started a family," and I had been told that he was dying.

After a series of tests it turned out that Albert has Raynaud's phenomenon, with some loops in his nails. He was prescribed different drugs and treatments: massage, laser, gymnastics, swimming, hydrotherapy. We were sent back home.

One year after our visit to Warsaw the lesion, already 10 cm in size, faded and almost completely disappeared. It left behind a strange scar and gray hairy skin. Now, even if we have to travel to the rheumatologist in

Olsztyn, everything is all right with the boy but my instinct does not let me feel that everything will be all right. I constantly hear the doctors' words in my head and wonder what else can I do for my son. He now has an insert in his right shoe to compensate for the shortness of the leg. I have made the insert for the entire foot, despite the doctor's advice to use a 1.5 cm insert only under the heel. I am afraid that every cough is not just a cold but will start the disease again. When my son is well behaved, I wonder if he is already ill.

Despite all my worries he is a normal boy who makes mischief at any time. He is scared of having blood taken so we do the blood tests every four or five months and not every month. The summer is coming so he will need a sun cream with a high protection again on his leg, and with low protection for the other leg so that both legs have similar color. He will again be able to swim in the lake every day.

In two years when he starts school, then maybe nobody will realize that he is different during sports lessons. His leg pains do not happen so often now; the skin after laser therapy is whiter and the hairs are lighter and finer. A cream makes his skin soft; playing scooter keeps his leg fit, bicycling helps joint mobility, swimming gives him pleasure and makes him fit and now he is very strong.

The Kangaroo ball is irreplaceable, and what Albert likes most is when he can apply the lotion on his leg. That is when he touches his little bones and says, "These are the bones of my body, this part is hard and this is soft." Recently he told a woman we know who has a six-month-old son that, "If Macius' also has a painful leg I will give him a cream to drive the pain away."

Scleroderma for me is something that causes my little son to wear an orthopedic shoe and makes him different from other boys. For Albert this is something that is natural and obvious and he pays it no attention. Only sometimes when he plays in the yard I can hear his friends asking: "Why do you have such leg?" and his answer: "Because this is my body and it has to be hard!"

♦ ❖ ♦

Judy Cowell
Daughter Alison, Linear Morphea
Missouri, USA

I am married and the mother of four children. Three months ago our oldest daughter, Alison, was diagnosed with linear morphea scleroderma; juvenile scleroderma.

Over the wintertime we noticed a large bruise-like mark over the lower part of her right buttock. She also had various patches that went down her right leg. They are ivory colored patches surrounded by a darker border.

We had gone to an adult dermatologist and he diagnosed her as having something completely different. I scheduled an appointment with the pediatric dermatologist who immediately knew what the mark was just by looking at it. It was biopsied and shown to be linear morphea scleroderma with a lot of inflammation.

We also had antinuclear antibody (ANA) and DNA titers drawn and they came back negative. Her course of therapy has been a topical ointment, an immunosuppressant, an antirheumatic, and an anti-inflammatory. If we see no improvement with these medications, I believe the next step is methotrexate.

My daughter, who is eight years old, has really done well with the medications and the whole diagnosis. We have been to an orthopedist for a baseline check of her symmetry and right now everything seems to be okay with her growth. We were told that if we can get her through her growth spurt with good growth she should do just fine.

◆ ❖ ◆

Kathy Parrish
Localized Scleroderma
Tennessee, USA

I am a forty-seven year old white female. I was diagnosed with focal or localized scleroderma, which is also known as juvenile scleroderma, at the age of eighteen months.

I spent a lot of my young life at the Children's Clinic at Vanderbilt Hospital in Nashville, Tennessee. I do not remember any of my treatment, but do have a report of my case that was included in *The Journal of Pediatrics* in March 1962.

Surgeries and skin grafts were done to loosen the tightness of my skin when I was very small. The disease affected the right side of my body. When I was young, I was fitted with a special shoe to lengthen my right leg in order for me to walk at a level pace. I was terrorized by other children at school who made stupid childish remarks about the special shoe, so eventually I stopped wearing it to avoid the harassment.

I married at the age of sixteen, and had my first child at the age of seventeen. I have two of the healthiest children that anyone could ever wish for. I am still married to the same man after thirty-one years.

I just lost my wonderful mother in 2001, and until now I never even thought of asking more questions of the past. I want to talk to more people about this disease and learn more about it.

Larella James
Son Cody, Morphea
Iowa, USA

Cody was diagnosed with morphea in October of 2001. He was eight at the time and had a white, leathery, hard patch developing under his right eye.

A year prior to Cody's diagnosis, I asked his pediatrician about a bruise under his eye that did not seem to want to go away. During another visit I asked about the bruise again, as it had turned into a white patch that then began to spread and harden. Both times I was told to put sunscreen on the patch.

Finally, during a checkup for my two year old, I asked the pediatrician to take one more look at Cody's patch. He did, and sent us to a specialist the very next day. I guess Cody needed more than sunscreen.

The specialist was a dermatologist. She took five minutes to give us a diagnosis and then sent us on our way. She advised us not to read anything about the disease because it would only scare us. We decided not to wait a year this time to see another doctor.

Cody has since been seen by a pediatric rheumatologist who confirmed the diagnosis. The doctor decided no treatment is warranted at this time. The jury is still out on this doctor, but he seems to know what he is talking about. We might give him a couple more months.

Since the diagnosis, my husband and I have been in overdrive trying to gain as much information as possible on the illness. Because it affects Cody's face we feel we need to be extremely proactive. Cody cannot cover up the scarring and he cannot hide from the stares or questions.

Along with educating ourselves, we have decided as a family to help empower our son. As adults, my husband and I feel an extreme lack of control over this situation. We can only imagine being a child who has to live with this illness. We decided that Cody needed to learn how to make decisions about his body. We all know he is going to have to make some tough ones very soon.

One of the first decisions Cody made, like most eight-year-old boys in 2002, was to dye his hair green. You should have seen the stylist's reaction when Cody jumped into the chair and said, "I want my hair green and my parents said it was my choice!"

She asked my husband, who was with Cody at the time, if he was a weekend dad. She did not want an angry mother coming in to the shop on Monday screaming about someone dyeing her son's hair green.

Shortly after the hair job, I found my son in the bathtub full of green water, crying. I knew it was serious when he did not scream the minute I opened the door and saw him naked. When I asked why he was crying he told me that his hair was not green anymore.

I brought him a mirror and assured him that it still was. He smiled when he looked in the mirror, a smile of such genuine relief that I began to cry.

He told me that since he had green hair no one at school had asked about his eye. No one had teased him about it, and he had not had to tell the kids he was contagious just so they would leave him alone.

Guess who was crying even harder after this conversation? I do not think I stopped for days. This was the first real conversation my son and I had had about his illness since his diagnosis.

That green hair turned out to be a miracle for us. He told me things after we left the bathroom that he had not ever before. We talked about the illness and how it might affect him. We talked about school, his future, and our love for him as a family, and mine for him as a mother.

I assured him that no matter what happens, we will always be there for him and he will always have the support of his family. I also assured him that he is strong enough to take what ever comes. Together, we are an unbeatable force.

It has been four months since Cody dyed his hair. It has faded and he has now decided he wants blue hair. I do not know if I am ready to battle the school system again but I have already made the hair appointment.

I am looking forward to a tub full of blue water and another "most meaningful" life conversation with my son.

◆ ❖ ◆

Mary-Charlotte
Linear
New York, USA

When I was five years old, I closed my finger in a lazy susan and a small brown spot appeared on my index finger. We all assumed that it was a bruise, as we had no reason to think otherwise. After a few weeks, the bruise was not going away, and my entire pointer finger was beginning to look slightly discolored. My parents took me to our pediatrician, and he took X rays and decided that it was just an infection. I took antibiotics for a couple of weeks but nothing changed.

I was then taken to a pediatric surgeon, who had no idea what it was. He recommended a dermatologist at Yale University Medical Center who diagnosed it as morphea. At that time, no treatment was prescribed or recommended, as morphea usually resolves itself after a couple of years.

For a second opinion, I was taken to a doctor in New York City. This doctor thought that a very different approach should be taken to control the disease. He prescribed intravenous methotrexate and steroids. My parents immediately decided against this treatment.

By this time, the brown markings had begun spreading up my hand and thumb, and onto my arm. After a year and a half, the disease had spread to my shoulder and upper back, causing muscle loss and discoloration. In some of the lesions, my skin was getting thicker and harder, while others stayed fairly soft. I was then diagnosed with linear, rather than morphea, juvenile scleroderma.

After visiting many doctors and having many tests in New York City, Pittsburgh, Connecticut, and New Jersey, I was taken to Boston to see a pediatric rheumatologist. While there, I had many tests that ended up being very helpful to the doctor. I first had an MRI, which was very difficult for me, as I was so afraid of it. In the end, the doctors had to anesthetize me in order to do the MRI. I also took a swallowing test, and a breathing test, as well as photographs, X rays, measurements, and blood work.

The doctor in Boston prescribed methotrexate. While the scleroderma did not ever make me ill, the methotrexate had very negative side affects. I was thin, pale and sickly. To reduce the side affects, I was given the medication through an injection once a week and had to have blood tests each week. This was when I was five to eight years old, and I had grown very afraid of needles, or being stuck by anything. I had a fear of all insects, because I thought that every bug was going to sting me.

When the spread of the scleroderma slowed, I began only taking methotrexate when the doctors suspected that it was active. If my arm was red or at all swollen, I was immediately put back on the methotrexate. At this point, I had begun seeing a doctor at the Hospital for Special Surgery in New York City. I was going to the hospital every week for occupational therapy, and every few weeks I also saw the doctor.

By this time I was in third grade, and although there is a lot I do not remember about my experience with scleroderma, there are several memories that stay in my mind. While going back and forth to hospitals, I became very scared of sick people and people in wheelchairs. I was afraid I would become like those sick people. I also grew very afraid of having surgery, especially when I began seeing the pediatric rheumatologist at the Hospital for Special *Surgery*. My mother says that she was happy that this was my main fear, because the doctors knew that surgery would not help cure the disease.

Having linear scleroderma was difficult because even when I felt healthy and normal, I had large brown marks on my skin that separated me from other children. The number of questions that I was asked, and that I am still asked today, hurt me in a way that none of my peers could understand. I had many stories about what the brown marks on my arm were, and none of them involved me being sick. Sometimes I said it was a scar, and sometimes just dirt from recess. These stories caused a problem when I had to miss school every week. Suddenly I realized that I could not tell people that I had to miss school because of the dirt on my arm.

I began telling some people the truth, but being young, and having immature friends, I got a lot of negative reactions. Some people thought scleroderma was contagious, and did not want to go near me. Other people treated me like I was dying. I did not want to be treated any differently, but some people could not understand that, and some people still do not understand that today.

I am now fourteen years old, and I have been in remission for about six years. I no longer take methotrexate or occupational therapy. I should probably still be taking occupational therapy, but I never seem to be able to continue it for very long, because none of the physical therapists understand that scleroderma is an ongoing problem, and I am not a patient who will ever be done with treatments.

Exercising at home is very important because I need to retain what little muscle and flexibility I still have in my arm, shoulder, and hand. I now see a doctor who is close to our house. She is a pediatric rheumatologist and she normally just takes measurements of my arm, and gives me a blood test to make sure that every thing is okay. We are no longer in search of a perfect doctor, because it seems with every doctor we see, we end up explaining what linear scleroderma is. We still hope that one day a new treatment will become available to scleroderma patients.

I enjoy horseback riding, and my family and I run a stable in our town. I do not play other sports, but I do not think I can really blame that on the linear scleroderma. My left side is significantly weaker than my right side, but I have learned to compensate for that. Although I am sure that I will never grow up to be a mountain climber, my life is not greatly affected by this weakness. I also love art, and playing the clarinet.

While I am older now, and no longer have to deal with people who think that scleroderma is contagious, the brown marks on my arm still bother me sometimes. When asked what happened to my arm, I normally just tell people it is a birthmark, until I feel that I can trust them to react the right way.

I still enjoy the comfort of wearing long sleeves in the winter, and feeling like I am just like everyone else, even though the marks on my arm have become a part of who I am today.

Up to this point in my life, I have yet to meet or speak to anyone who has scleroderma. I pray for everyone who is faced with scleroderma, and hope that soon there will be a cure for this rare disease.

Update – March 2004

Scleroderma has proven once again that it is an unpredictable and often uncontrollable force. My years of remission left me feeling positive that scleroderma was nearly out of my life for good. While there were still doctor appointments, routine blood work, some physical therapy, and questions from curious peers, it was no longer active, and this made all the difference.

It amazes me how quickly one can adapt to change, so long as it is for the better. While I was in remission, I forgot what it was like to be actively treating an incurable disease. I forgot what it was to feel sick and drained. I forgot, for a time, what it was to feel different.

Throughout my freshman year of high school it seemed that my health was deteriorating. I felt very weak and often developed colds and other illnesses. Every doctor I saw denied that scleroderma in its active state causes illness, so I assumed it was just allergies.

In mid-August, the summer before my sophomore year, routine blood work revealed abnormalities. My sedimentation rate was above normal. This was also the case when I was younger and the disease entered an active state. I was very worried about these results, although everyone assured me that it was a mistake. I was always told that once scleroderma was in remission for many years, it would not come back.

A week before my first day of school, I left my rheumatologist with the news that the disease was active again. I was immediately told to start taking prednisone and methotrexate. This was one of the scariest times of my life. Everything happened so quickly. One day I was just a normal fifteen year old, then all of the sudden I was sick again.

The earliest days of treatment were the most difficult. Adjusting to the steroids was not easy. I was left feeling sick and weak. The first week of methotrexate was not very difficult, but by the second dose it began making me very ill. School began, and keeping up with my work became my goal. Every day was a struggle. Months passed and I slowly grew more used to the medicine. Unfortunately, it was not having a strong enough effect on the disease, so it had to be increased, therefore I started methotrexate injections.

Now I am trying to wean myself off of steroids. It is a very difficult process, and has made me feel sick, but it is worth it. Being off the steroids will be a huge hurdle in fighting scleroderma.

While there is no stopping the spread and activity of scleroderma, I still hope the medicine will work and my life will return to normal. With the help of my friends and doctors, I know we can eventually beat this for good.

◆ ❖ ◆

Meghann
Morphea
California, USA

I am sixteen now and have had morphea for about two to three years. When I first started to develop small red spots on my stomach, I thought it was just a rash. When they got bigger, I thought it was ringworm.

I finally went to the doctor. They gave me some antifungal creams and referred me to another doctor's name because they did not know what it was.

I went to that doctor, and she took a biopsy. She called me back about a week later and told me I have morphea. I was very sad to hear that the spots would never go away, but at least new ones might be prevented.

I cried for about a week. By this time they were getting bigger, about the size of a tennis ball. I should be going to a dermatologist now to keep track of the sizes, but since I am only sixteen and my dad has no time to take me, I am just sitting and watching them get bigger.

I have about five or six spots. One of them is very hard and yellow. When I go out I put a bandage over it and if anyone asks about the other ones, I tell them they are bruises. I am afraid to tell anyone that it is morphea, because it sounds so gross.

I am getting more and more afraid that they will spread. But I have to say I am getting more comfortable with them. It does not bother me as much when I look in the mirror, so I am back to wearing a bathing suit. I have just accepted that they are there and that I cannot do anything about it.

Melanie Weisbecker
Linear Morphea
New York, USA

I am eighteen years old and have been diagnosed with linear morphea for two and a half years.

It started as a small white patch on my neck. It soon grew up my neck, and I have lost hair in that spot. I have brown and white patches of skin all over my upper back. I am self-conscious of it, so I will not wear my hair up, or wear little tank tops.

My doctor says there is no treatment and that my scars will be there forever. I hate that feeling. The only good thing about this disease is that it makes you a better person. I am modest about myself and am greatful for what I have.

I am also thankful that these are the only morphea patches I have gotten, because a lot of people have it worse.

CHAPTER 6

Localized Scleroderma
Linear and Morphea

*Now I am in the process of trying to find a doctor,
a sensitive one, who is willing to help me even though
it is not a disease that will kill me.*

—Tami

Introduction
Developing Empathy: A Researcher's Perspective on Being Diagnosed with Scleroderma
by Vanessa L. Malcarne, Ph.D.

Dr. Vanessa Malcarne is Professor, Department of Psychology at San Diego State University. She received her PhD in clinical psychology from the University of Vermont in 1989. Her research focuses on quality of life for people with cancer and rheumatic diseases (including scleroderma). She also studies the effects of chronic illness on spouses and children.

In clinical psychology, my field of study and work, people have asked me many times if it matters if a therapist has personal experience with the problems they are treating.

For example, is a therapist better at helping people with alcohol problems if the therapist has also struggled with and overcome similar issues, or does that make the therapist too biased, unable to appreciate what might be different about another person's experience? Or, is it better for a marital therapist to have struggled with marital problems him/herself, or instead preferable for them to have achieved a happy marriage?

There is no easy answer to this question, and there are successful therapists from all walks of lives. However, there is no question that having personal experience with a problem changes one's perspective. This was very true for me with regards to scleroderma.

In the late 1980s, I was in the middle of my doctoral studies in clinical psychology at the University of Vermont, preparing for a career in research and teaching. The focus of my research was how people adapt to cancer diagnoses—indeed, the focus of my dissertation was how patients cope with learning that they have cancer. I conducted in-depth interviews with cancer patients and their family members, trying to come to a deeper understanding of how devastating news about a threat to one's health—and life—affects an individual's personal life, as well as their family.

I was twenty-eight at the time, and frankly my capacity for empathy with the persons I studied was somewhat limited, because I had never experienced serious illness myself. I had never had anything other than a cold or flu, or an occasional upset stomach—indeed, I had never even been treated at a hospital or clinic.

Toward the end of my third year in graduate school, I noticed one morning that a section of my skin had turned completely white. Now, I'm quite light in complexion anyway, and this was in Vermont, where after a long winter indoors many of us look quite pasty!

However, I could tell right away that something was unusual, and I called the student health clinic for an appointment, wondering if I was perhaps having some sort of allergic reaction to something. The physician's assistant at the student health clinic couldn't figure out what was causing the skin to change color, and actually asked if perhaps I had visited a tanning salon recently and had inadvertently covered part of my body with a towel! (Believe me, tanning salons weren't common in Vermont in the mid-1980s.) I was referred to a dermatologist for follow-up.

A couple of days later, on a Friday afternoon, I visited the dermatologist, still assuming I was having some sort of allergic reaction, and not particularly concerned about the situation. The dermatologist took a rather quick look at my white skin and said, "You either have scleroderma or breast cancer."

I said, in what I've since learned is the typical response of scleroderma patients learning their diagnosis, "Sclero *what?*"

The dermatologist responded, "It's a severe rheumatic disease that will cause your skin to become like leather and can be fatal. We'll do a biopsy, and get back to you in a few days." That was my introduction to scleroderma—and to receiving bad medical news. I don't even remember the biopsy, and don't think I said another thing to either the doctor or nurse during the rest of the appointment.

I went downstairs and sat in the lobby for about an hour, unsure what to do next, but feeling that my life had, in an instant, completely changed. My confidence that I had control over my health evaporated.

I felt terrified, helpless, and alone. I called my husband, but couldn't seem to tell him what had happened on the phone—the words wouldn't come out. So, rather than trying to explain things over the telephone, I asked him to come pick me up at the hospital. He was an hour away, so I had plenty of time to sit in the lobby and think about what had happened, and what I was going to do next.

I remember, as I sat in the lobby, thinking about how ironic it was that, after years of studying how people respond to diagnoses of serious, potentially fatal illness, I had myself just had the same experience. The researcher in me recognized that this was a great opportunity to observe, first-hand, exactly how a dignosis could affect someone!

I personally understood for the first time how completely overwhelming the experience was, and how difficult to put into words. I felt the panic, the fear, the uncertainty. I wondered, How will I tell my husband? My parents? My friends? What will I tell them?

As I sat and processed what had happened, it occurred to me that I hadn't even asked the doctor any questions, and that the whole experience, after his words about breast cancer or scleroderma, seemed like a blur. I also had the sense that I was at the beginning of a medical journey, and that there were many different paths that the journey could take.

Part of my research has always focused on coping strategies—what do people do to cope with stress, such as that presented by a diagnosis of serious illness, and do some coping strategies work better than others? I had read lots of scholarly articles on this subject, arguing that this type of coping worked best, and that type of coping didn't work at all—and I realized I was about to learn for myself whether the "experts" knew what they were talking about!

My first challenge was to get through the next four days, until I would learn the results of my biopsy. Remember that I was a graduate student, and what do graduate students do to address any and all problems? They go to the library and read!

So that's what I did. The next day, I went to the medical school library, and looked up everything I could find about scleroderma. I already knew quite a bit about breast cancer from my work with cancer patients, and was actually pretty sure that my symptoms did not match that. Rather, I was more curious about this disease that I had never heard of before.

I quickly learned that scleroderma was a serious but poorly understood disease that mainly affected women of middle age (I was a bit on the young side). I also learned that there were many different subtypes.

I read and read, and took lots of notes, and made lots of photocopies of articles and chapters, and after two full days in the library I felt much more educated, and more prepared to successfully manage scleroderma, if that's what I had.

And interestingly, I was fairly confident by this point of what my actual diagnosis would be. I was quite certain that I had morphea—a type of localized scleroderma that is characterized by thickened and tightened skin plaques. This is one of the least serious variants of scleroderma, so this was very encouraging to me.

The next Tuesday, I went back to get the results of my biopsy. The dermatologist told me that I did have scleroderma, and that the biopsy had confirmed this. I told him that I had spent the weekend reading at the medical school library, and that I wasn't surprised as it seems that my skin condition exactly matched the presentation of morphea.

And here was another point in the process in which I experienced first-hand what many of the cancer patients I had interviewed had told me about—my physician scolded me for trying to learn more about scleroderma!

He told me that he discouraged his patients from reading too much about their condition, especially in medical books and journals, because he found that it just frightened people and that they couldn't really understand the information anyway. I had always been surprised when cancer patients had told me that their oncologists discouraged them from seeking second opinions or additional information, and now I was experiencing the same thing.

And actually my experience had been the opposite of what the doctor thought it would be. Going to the library and reading had proved to be an excellent coping strategy for me, because it made me feel more in control, decreased my anxiety, passed the time while I was waiting for the biopsy results, and helped me figure out what questions I wanted to ask when I received the diagnosis.

Research on coping has found that there are two kinds of people: information-seekers and information-avoiders. I've always been an information seeker; having lots of information makes me feel better, and thus I spent my weekend in the library. For other people, it might have been better to take a trip, spend time with family, go to the movies—in other words, using distraction to avoid thinking about the upcoming medical appointment.

This probably wouldn't have worked for me, but it was another example of how actually experiencing a serious diagnosis helped me toward a greater understanding of what the experience was all about. I realized that there was no right or wrong way of coping—the question was not what type of coping worked in general, but what type of coping worked for a particular individual, at a particular point in time.

At the time I was diagnosed, in the mid 1980s, less was known about the relationship between localized scleroderma and the limited and diffuse types of the disease. Some doctors thought that localized scleroderma might be the early stages of the more severe versions.

I lived with the fear that my morphea might develop into something much more serious for several years, until I was seen by a rheumatologist in California who told me that would not happen. And this was when I learned another important lesson about coping with a serious diagnosis, that I have since repeated to hundreds of scleroderma patients, at meetings and conferences and in personal encounters: Get treatment from an expert!

My dermatologist in Vermont meant well, and I'm still impressed with how quickly he diagnosed me—I've heard dozens of stories of people who waited years for a definite diagnosis—but he had never treated a scleroderma patient before, and didn't really know much about the disease. Thus, he couldn't teach me much about it, and also didn't know much about treatment options. I went untreated and wondered for three years whether I would suddenly find myself with a more advanced form of the disease. When I finally was treated by specialist in rheumatology, with extensive experience with scleroderma of all types, I felt tremendous relief, as I knew that I was in the most capable hands possible.

I've been lucky. I still have morphea but my condition never got any worse, and it never affected my health in any other way, or my ability to do the things I want to do. Interestingly, finding that white patch of skin was one of the most important things that ever happened to me. Receiving a diagnosis of scleroderma helped me grow as a psychologist and a researcher, as well as personally.

The experience helped me to develop greater empathy with the patients I worked with and studied, and to have a deeper and truer appreciation for the magnitude of what they were facing.

It also led me to expand my research focus beyond cancer to include scleroderma, and I've been privileged for the past decade to learn from scleroderma patients and their families, and to pass that information on through articles and presentations to other patients and their families.

◆❖◆

Audley Blythe Loewen
Louisiana, USA

Our twenty-one year old daughter, Diana, was diagnosed in August of 1999 with morphea scleroderma. Since it is on her face and head, she is considered to have the en coup de sabre type of morphea.

After one diagnosis of vitiligo, my motherly intuition told me that the diagnosis was not correct, so we made appointments with two more doctors who confirmed the morphea diagnosis. One did a biopsy.

We found a doctor in Birmingham, Alabama, Dr. Craig Elmets, who specializes in scleroderma, and he used a UVA1 light on Diana's lesions for approximately six months. She has shown no signs of the disease progressing.

She is a very happy and beautiful girl and covers her scar with Dermablend, which is a corrective cosmetic. Since the one scar on her forehead is en coup de sabre, it is indented so her skin is uneven there. She deals with it wonderfully. The area on her scalp is right at her part-line and because she has lost hair in that area, she parts her hair on the opposite side and it looks fine.

Joanne Grow
New Jersey, USA

I was diagnosed with morphea and linear scleroderma about two years ago. After having Mohs surgery performed to remove some facial skin cancer, I decided to look at my back in the mirror and noticed areas that were white and encircled by an outer lavender ring. In hindsight, my scleroderma probably started nearly ten years ago in a very gradual and quiet way.

First was a stage of gradual inflammation followed by eventual, unrelenting fatigue. As in many cases, it was easy to ignore a little weight gain and to blame my fatigue on a very active career in technical writing for some major corporations. Following one more trip to the dermatologist for yet another biopsy, I learned that I had this autoimmune disease. One lesion led to multiple lesions.

In a two-year period, the scleroderma has gained some ground. I now have multiple lesions on my back, a linear strip on my stomach, and multiple lesions on my face and neck. I have what I call "active periods" when I do get a little tired. The lesion that stretches from my cheek, around my mouth and down my chin, slightly affects my speech. The rest of the lesions join in their own special way!

I participate in fundraising walks for scleroderma research, and I volunteer for the International Scleroderma Network. The way I look at it all now is that it has just impacted my body, not my heart or mind.

◆❖◆

Kathleen A. Perman
Wisconsin, USA

I am fifty-eight years young. I am a mother of three and grandmother of five, soon to be six. I have lived in Wisconsin all my life. I have been through a lot of things and really do not know whether there is a connection among any of them.

I was diagnosed with localized scleroderma when I was six months pregnant with my son in 1965. It started with blotches on my right arm. After the delivery in December, I discovered that all the symptoms went directly to my left arm and stayed on that side of my body. Then it spread in clusters to my right leg, my stomach, and under both arms near my breasts.

Over the years a lot of it has cleared up, except my left arm looks like it belongs on a different person's body. There is no muscle form to it and I am limited in doing exercise with my left arm. My fingers were really stiff until my chiropractor performed manipulations to my back and hand in 1966-1967.

I have lived with scleroderma as it is for many years and just dealt with it. I went through a lot of traumatic events in my life. I started getting really sick and weak in 1993-1994 and after a lot of intensive testing, I was found to have celiac disease. That meant eliminating wheat, rye, oats and barley from my diet. That was quite a challenge, but I found I did feel better when I changed my diet.

Around 1998 through 2001, I became very ill again. I reached the point where I could not work anymore in 2000, and I went on disability. Again I had a lot of testing by numerous doctors.

The doctor who had diagnosed me with celiac disease finally found that my liver was damaged to the point that the only thing that would save me would be a liver transplant. She introduced me to the University of Wisconsin Transplant Department. I went through intensive testing again to make sure that I was healthy enough to be deserving of a transplant. Thankfully I was, but had to wait like everyone else.

My health got so bad that I was admitted to the hospital because my significant other could not deal with me any longer. I do not even remember all of the year 2000. The doctors told him at that point that I would never go home. But thanks to a miracle, I received a new liver from a wonderful person named Stephen. I was in surgery for seventeen hours. It took a long time for recovery. I spent some time in a nursing home to learn how to walk again.

I am going to celebrate my new life on November 02, 2002, when it will be two wonderful years since my transplant. I am so happy to be alive and living so well. But there are still so many unanswered questions for me. My doctors are telling me that scleroderma is no longer a problem for me. I just would like to have some answers as to what brought up all of the conditions that I have dealt with most of my life. No one else in my family has had these things.

The transplant team said they will probably never know for sure why my liver became damaged. I would just like to know if scleroderma was the cause of my health problems, or does it just go away? I have an appointment with my transplant team next week so I hope to ask them a lot of questions again. I want some answers but I also want the doctors to come up with something soon that will help so many of us who are dealing with the problems of scleroderma.

Where does it start and where does it go after that? Does it ever end?

Update – November 2002

Last Friday I had a deep Doppler ultrasound and liver biopsy. The tests showed that I am going through a mild liver rejection due to my immune system getting screwed up.

Naturally I wondered what I had done wrong. My wonderful doctor reassured me that I have been doing everything right. It is just something that can happen with my weakened immune system. So I have been put on megadoses of prednisone for three days and will taper down after that. I had been off that dreaded drug for over a year now and was feeling so great. But here I go again, flying higher than a kite. I feel like a cat on a hot tin roof. The side effects to this medicine are not pleasant, but you *gotta* do what you *gotta* do.

I would never want to go through a transplant again, even if I were to reject the one that I was blessed to receive in 2000. I also do not know if I would get the opportunity again since there are so many others on the waiting list now.

But anyway, I did not get an opportunity to talk to my doctor about the scleroderma, celiac disease or other immune problems. I really want to know if there is a connection to all of this.

After I get through with this rejection episode, and I will, I need to find someone who will really let me know what is going on with my body. I know I probably will not be able to change any of it, but I would like to know if any of this will be passed on to my children or darling grandchildren, and if there is anything that I personally can do to help them with advice in advance.

I have a sister with multiple sclerosis, so immune problems run in the family. My mother, who passed away in 1992, had a lot of the same symptoms that I have now with celiac disease. My mother's doctors never told her anything about her health problems either.

I have an appointment with the transplant doctors again soon and I hope to get some serious advice from them, or hopefully they can suggest someone who can help me further.

Tammy M.
California, USA

Although I cannot remember what it was like, there was a time when I did not have scleroderma. When I was eleven I was involved in an all terrain vehicle (ATV) accident. My foot got caught between the tire and the fender and it ripped up the side of my ankle pretty bad. We were out in the desert, so the wound was full of sand and eventually ended up getting infected. But it healed up, or so I thought.

A few months later, I dropped a one pound bottle of hair conditioner, cap first, on the instep of my foot on the same leg. That formed a rather large bruise, which faded to a purplish scar.

Several months later, those two wounds kind of joined together in a linear fashion and began traveling up my leg. It looked like a rope or a braid on the back of my leg. I lost a lot of flexibility in that leg.

After a year of doctors with blank faces and no answers (which enraged me for at least the next ten years) my mom and I happened upon someone who actually knew what I had and she diagnosed me with linear scleroderma. I took medication for it for awhile, but being an angry teenager at the time, I was not a very good patient.

For much of my adult life I have lived with some form of denial and have not been actively seeking treatment. Unfortunately, the scarring is continuing to progress, albeit slowly.

I now have some lesions on my tailbone and spine that are beginning to concern me. The skin is so thin on my tailbone and there are no fat deposits, so sitting has become quite uncomfortable. Within the last six months I have also developed vitiligo.

After seventeen years of dealing with scleroderma and somehow getting through the tortures of adolescence relatively unscathed, the vitiligo has brought out many of my insecurities and fears. I jokingly say, "I now have spots to go with my stripes!" But all joking aside, I am approaching a point where I think I am ready to start fighting this on a variety of levels.

When I was first diagnosed there was no such thing as the Internet. I always felt that my family and I were the only ones in the world who knew what scleroderma was.

Now I am in the process of trying to find a doctor, a sensitive one who is willing to help me, even though it is not a disease that will kill me. I may see a nutritionist and a physical therapist, and maybe even a therapist to start talking about all the things I never dealt with because being in denial was the only way I could cope.

Anna Bason
Alabama, USA

My morphea started as bruise-like marks on the backs of my legs about three years ago, after I had just fought cervical cancer and won! At first my family and I thought that they were only bruises and that I might be diabetic. When I went to the doctor she thought it might be morphea, but the test results showed something else. After a year wait to see a skin doctor, I was finally told that it was morphea. I was told there was no known cure or treatment, but I was put on a steroid ointment.

At my next visit my doctor informed me that I could not be in extremely cold climates. This broke my heart. I grew up in central New York and moved to Alabama to work. I thought I could never again see a white Christmas with my family that still lives in New York, or go sledding with my son, or have a snowball fight with him, or even build a snowman. However, I have since found out that Raynaud's is mostly associated with systemic scleroderma, not morphea, and that even if I had Raynaud's, I could still do all these things; I would just have to dress warmly.

The marks cover most of the back of my legs. They are also under my left arm, and on both breasts, my left foot, and shoulder. When people ask me what the marks are I explain that I have morphea and I tell them what I know. I have had people ask if my husband beats me, or if I am accident-prone.

I live each day to the fullest and hope that as I spread understanding of morphea to the people around me, it will make it easier for the next person they may encounter who has morphea. With my faith, I know that if I can beat cancer, I can beat this too!

Becky
Illinois, USA

I am a forty-two-year-old mother of two teens, and have been married for twenty years.

I was finally diagnosed with fibromyalgia in 1998, myofascial pain syndrome and osteoarthritis in 2001, and just recently found out that I have mitral valve prolapse.

I have what appears to be a bruise on the inside of my forearm. I also have what looks like an inflamed vein coming out of the bruise.

My primary care physician referred me to a dermatologist, who took one look at the bruise and said that he was sure it was morphea. A biopsy was taken, along with blood work to see if this condition is systemic.

At first I was so upset. I felt betrayed by my body. I am a very health-minded person, and am really angry that my body appears to be attacking itself.

I will get the results of the testing in two weeks, but the doctor seemed very sure of his diagnosis. The muscle in my forearm has already atrophied, and it has only been four weeks!

Thank goodness for my wonderful husband and sons, as they seem to be taking it all in stride. I have a very upbeat attitude, and will just take things as they come, trying to keep the blues away.

As always, keep your chin up, we can handle this!

Beth
Texas, USA

My story began when I was six years old and continues today at age thirty-six. My first morphea spot appeared on my left shin. It was about the size of a dime and grew to the size of an oval silver dollar. My mother took me to the doctor and he said it was a bruise that never healed.

We didn't think anything more about it until I was ten, when my mother asked me who had been grabbing me around the waist. My waist and my lower back had red marks like I had been squeezed.

Soon after the marks started to enlarge and change shape and they took on a different color. My mother took me to a dermatologist and I was told that I had very dry skin.

These spots went through several stages of activity. They first had a reddish purple ring around the oval and the center was white and scaly. Then, when the activity stopped, the reddish ring darkened to brown like a scar while the center stayed white, but not scaly.

Later on when I was a teenager I went to another dermatologist to see what they had to say. I was told I had morphea but they did not know much about it and could not tell me anything about it other than what they had read about it.

I went on for years explaining to every doctor that I have ever had to see for regular medical visits that I am not being beaten by anyone. I inform them that I have morphea, which is some kind of rare skin disease.

When I had my first child I was very scared that this would be something I would pass on to my child. My doctor assured me this was not something hereditary. As my stomach grew the spots did not change at all. I had my first child at age nineteen, and another at age twenty-one.

All these years I never had any new spots appear until I had my third child at age twenty-nine. All of a sudden, several months after that birth, my back, sides and stomach had all new spots and these varied in size from a dime to a six-inch oval.

I was horrified. Why were these things coming back all of a sudden? What triggered them to appear, and this time, in such a mass quantity?

I went to my family doctor and he said he thought I might have scleroderma. So he sent me to see another dermatologist. This dermatologist was familiar with morphea and actually had another patient with it but not to the same degree as mine.

He put me on a medication which is used for acne and he said studies had been done that proved this medication would stop the spot's activity and make them dormant. I took the medication for six months and the spots seemed to have finished their cycle, but I do not think it was the medication. I think they just ran their course.

Within a few years, more new ones started appearing all the time; however, these are not really large ones. They are about the size of a quarter or smaller. Some of them do not have the oval shape or the white middle. They are dark brown, bruise-like spots.

What seems weird is that they seem to be in areas that get pressure trauma. For example, one day I was carrying a grocery-shopping basket on my arm between my wrist and elbow and the basket was heavy. The next day or so I noticed marks on my arm. The doctor said that has nothing to do with it.

My spots are mostly on my trunk. I also have little brown ones on my chest by my arm where my bra strap lies, and all over my back, and the same old one on my leg shin.

I haven't been too upset about these, mainly because my clothes cover them. What really got me sparked to search for information is because my oldest daughter has had one spot on her ankle since she was ten. That spot has grown to be about six inches long and it is very dark brown.

At that time, our family doctor said it was the same thing I have. We did not believe it because it did not have any of the characteristics of my spots.

She is eighteen now, and this spot has grown from two inches when she was ten, to six inches, and it really bothers her because it is very noticeable. I looked at it the other day and it now has similar characteristics of the oval shape with a darker ring. I feel sorry for her because I sure would hate to see her start getting these all over her body.

I am very excited to know that there are so many people who have this same thing. It is nice to hear familiar stories. Now I do not feel like such a freak, as my dad used to tell me I could join the circus and be in a side show as the spotted girl.

❖ ❖ ❖

Brenda J. Kelly
Michigan, USA

I was diagnosed with morphea scleroderma about twelve years ago. It started with a dark linear mark on my lower back that is still there, and then with a pure white circle on my cheek.

The skin on these areas was very taut and dry feeling. Although the texture is better now, which may be due to the lotion I use, the spot on my face is not pure white any more. It is a different color than the rest of my face.

This year it has changed. I went to a dermatologist and he said it is just deterioration. *Just?*

It is continuing to deteriorate, and I am afraid it is affecting my eye because the eyes are held in place by tissue. Friends have started noticing this a little. Luckily I wear glasses, but I am getting more self-conscious.

I will be seeing a doctor soon and hopefully he will be able to help. I just wanted to share with others. Although I know my case is not serious or life threatening, it is my story and it concerns me.

Cara Chiarappa
California, USA

I was diagnosed with morphea when I was eighteen years old. I am now thirty-one.

My first spot was on my upper back and it has very slowly spread to my left arm, abdomen, left upper leg, and right lower leg. Over the years I struggled with my ugly skin. But I have come to accept it.

I tried one medication, but it made me so nauseated that I stopped. I also remember using some steroid cream, but it did not seem to help. So I basically just lived with it.

I fell in love with and married a wonderful man who loves me as I am. I am now four months pregnant. Over the last six months my right hand has become swollen and tight, and both of my knees are stiff and sore. My latest spot is on the top of my left hand.

Until now I had only seen a dermatologist, but I recently saw a rheumatologist who says it is limited or localized scleroderma. Because of the pregnancy I cannot start any treatment like methotrexate, but I read a story about some homeopathic treatments, and I would be open to that.

Carla M.
Minnesota, USA

I am a twenty-nine-year-old mother of three. I have localized morphea on my lower back.

It first appeared when I was in junior high, and has grown slowly since then. It started out as a spot on my back that looked just like a bruise that would not go away, and it was accompanied by lower back pain. It now spans from one side of me to the other, with one main lesion in the center, which branches out and has other spots around it.

It still looks just like a bruise, and if people see it they usually gasp and say, "What happened?" Luckily, it's not difficult to hide it, since it is on my back.

Most of the time I don't even think about it. It is not life threatening, but mostly is just an annoyance. But I am fearful that it could spread to other areas.

I was diagnosed early on, but have never had any treatments. I would really like to stop it from getting any larger. Does any one know of successful treatments for this type of morphea?

For a long time I have felt like somewhat of a freak, and did not even think about searching on the Internet about it until recently. I would love to talk with others who have similar morphea conditions.

Francisco
Bogota, Colombia

This story was translated from Spanish to English by Edwin Lamoli-Torres, who is a retired professor from the University of Puerto Rico at Mayaguez. The Spanish version of this story is in Chapter 9.

Fifteen days ago, I was diagnosed with morphea scleroderma. I first noticed the presence of the disease when I began to see red blemishes on the trunk of my body, which later began to get hard and brittle, resembling scars.

I have found differences in the size of the blemishes on my back, a thigh, an arm, a hand, a foot and my waist; all on the left side of my body.

I feel distressed with the diagnosis, since the dermatologist told me that the disease is chronic and that the treatment will have to go on for years. At present, I have been prescribed a medication and an ointment to be applied to the blemishes.

I would be very grateful for any information on this subject and I am at your disposal to offer any help that you may need. Please, feel free to write me, whenever you wish.

◆ ❖ ◆

Kelli Miller
Texas, USA

I am a twenty-six year old, married mother of two girls. I was diagnosed with morphea in the first grade. When my mother first noticed the spots she thought someone at school was hitting me! But when they did not go away she contacted the family doctor.

Since then I have seen over forty doctors related to this. The spots have continued to spread over my abdomen and my back. In the past few years they have spread to my upper arm and are progressing downward.

I have had many medications prescribed. Anywhere from drinking Potaba six times a day to applying a topical ointment and wrapping my abdomen in plastic wrap overnight—talk about uncomfortable!

No one has ever done blood work or biopsied the affected areas and this makes me wonder how they're so sure this is only a "cosmetic" disease. Only lately have I thought my chest pains might be related. We have only seen doctors in the Houston area, so they have all been dumbfounded by the spots.

Going through school I hated having to change clothes in gym class. A snooty girl one time called attention to them by saying, "Oh, what a cool bathing suit you must have, with all of those holes in it." I guess she thought they were tan lines! I just said yes and changed my clothes as fast as I could.

I have not given much thought to it, because my husband is the only person who sees the spots, and he accepts and loves me the way I am. Now that I have gotten a spot on my upper chest and one on my leg, I am getting a bit nervous. I would like to find something that will keep these silly things from spreading to my face.

On December 10, 2000, I went to my rheumatologist appointment. She confirmed the morphea diagnosis. She says it is not internal and since I have had it for twenty years, there is very little chance of it crossing over. I will be starting cosmetology school in January, and the vain side of me wanted to know if we could lighten up the spots that cannot be covered by clothing.

Update – June 2002

I want to sound upbeat about all of this, but I feel helpless. I have since finished my education and am now a licensed cosmetologist. But that is not to say it was an easy road I traveled.

I have had hand surgery for a trigger finger, and surgery on my foot for heel spurs and nerve tumors. This was during the middle part of my beauty school. When I started trying to walk again, I had running refills on painkillers and several electric massage therapy sessions, but the pain was not gone!

Because of the foot problems, my doctor said it would be best to lose some weight. He said this in a very positive, "Please do not hit me," kind of voice. I guess fatigue had caused me to put on a few unnoticed pounds, although I was the only one who did not notice them. In the last six months, I have lost forty pounds, and this has helped me get off the painkillers.

I have not kept up on seeing my rheumatologist. But I have to travel two hours to the city of Houston, and find parking in the medical center, just to have someone me, "Yep, you still have it, and no, we have not found a cure!" That does not make a cheerful ride home for me, and I have been told to keep my stress levels down, to not aggravate the disease.

I still get chest pains, and my family doctor says they are bones rubbing together. I have trouble breathing when the pains strike. I can only take very shallow breaths. And they just come and go, with no rhyme or reason.

My husband says I should go to another doctor for a second opinion, but I am scared witless of what they might have to say. I want the physical pain to go away, but I also do not want the emotional pain.

I live my life everyday like an "average Joe." If I let it, it could bring me down quickly. But when I feel like I am heading in that direction, I just take a look at my beautiful gifts I have been given, Madison and Morgan. And I am thankful that I am still here another day. Things could be a lot worse!

◆ ❖ ◆

Lama
Dubai, United Arab Emirates (UAE)

I never thought of sharing my story, but after reading the other stories I was really touched and found the courage to write about my own experience. I am twenty years old and I was only eighteen when the whole thing started. My mom noticed a small spot on my back, but we did not think it was anything important. But I was worried when it started getting larger and darker in color.

Naturally, I hoped that it would not appear somewhere where other people might notice it. I became very worried when a similar spot appeared on my thigh, and another one next to my knee.

I went to many doctors and I hated them all because I wanted to hear something positive and did not want to be disappointed. All the doctors told me that it is clear that what I have is morphea.

They did many tests to check that the morphea would not develop into something major. They told me I do not need to worry a lot about it.

I tried a lot of medicines but nothing worked. I got very depressed and could not talk about it to anyone. The only people who knew about it were my family. None of my friends ever saw the spots.

One of the things that I really worried about was my boyfriend. I was really terrified that he might get disgusted by the way the spots looked. One day when I was really depressed, I got the courage to tell him.

I was shocked at how easy he took it. It felt great having someone know about it and not think that it is a weird thing. I know the spots are very noticeable, but he acted as if they were invisible and he kept saying that no one would notice them. I know he was saying this because he wants to make me feel better—and he did!

What I am trying to say is that I really got over my severe depression with help from my boyfriend. It makes me feel great to know that he wants to marry me and spend the rest of his life with me, as if these spots were not bothering him at all.

I want to know about any treatments for morphea, because I still cry myself to sleep sometimes when I think about it. I worry all the time that a similar spot might appear on my face or on a place that I cannot hide. Just thinking about that possibility depresses me.

◆❖◆

Maria Clemente
Italy

*This story was translated from Italian to English by Kevin Howell. He is
a Clinical Scientist for Professor Black at the Royal Free Hospital in London.
The Italian version of this story is in Chapter 10.*

My morphea was diagnosed in 1998, although my first tests were done
about two years before at one of Italy's best dermatology hospitals after
some signs of the disease appeared.

I think, on the basis of information that I have collected, that the onset
of my disease was closely related to a long period of insomnia and stress,
caused by the pain in my ribs due to osteoporosis.

At first a pearly mark about the size of a coin appeared at the center
of my back, between the shoulder blades. The lesion had a reddish edge
of around five millimeters.

Then the mark started to extend until it reached a diameter of about
seven centimeters, with hardening and indentation of the area of involved
skin. Further small marks appeared on my forearms and legs, this time dark
and with a slight indentation.

From various tests including histopathology of a skin biopsy, oesoph-
ageal manometry, as well as lung function, only a slight respiratory failure
came to light. It is possible anyway, that this finding is the result of an episode
of pneumonia diagnosed when I was younger. However, no involvement
at a systemic level was found.

I think that the major damage has been to my eyesight, presenting
as a sudden deterioration in the function of my eyes as the disease has
developed.

I would like an opinion on the eventual course of the disease, and also
some advice on how I should deal with my form of scleroderma.

◆ ❖ ◆

Michelle (JR)
California, USA

My life took a large turn six months ago. I am still trying to sort through the pieces of a puzzle I never knew I was supposed to keep the pieces to. To put it plainly and simply, I am swimming in a deep sea of confusion and real frustration.

In September 2001, I suffered from a horrible sunburn. Like any other sunburn, the pain and the peeling went away and my life went back to normal.

In April 2002, I was lying in bed one night and I noticed that there was a part of my arm where it felt like something hard was underneath my skin. I thought it was odd, yet forgot about it until a week later, when the spot turned a blotchy white.

The spot covered roughly a square inch on my outer bicep. Figuring it was just from sun or a rash, I put some antibiotic cream on it and ignored it. A month went by with no change and I became concerned because the white patch now looked like shiny scar tissue and it was as thick as leather. It was now beginning to itch as well.

Everyone who looked at it was baffled and I thought that was never a good sign, so I made an appointment with my doctor.

Living in a small town, my doctor had never seen anything like this, and prescribed some cortisone cream assuming it was a fungus and it would disappear in a week. When it remained unchanged they decided to take a skin biopsy that left me with a large purple circle on my arm, and they determined it was morphea scleroderma.

I had never heard of morphea scleroderma, so I searched the Internet and bookstores, and much to my dismay I learned that it is a very rare skin disease that no one really knows much about.

I had my first appointment with a dermatologist today. He prescribed a new cream, which seems to have helped decrease the size by thirty percent for his one other patient who has been struggling with this for five years. Apparently my insurance company does not find it important enough to cover medication for this unimportant disease for a few rare freaks, or at least that is how I felt when they denied coverage.

I had been looking forward to this appointment, expecting I could ask all my questions and receive a few answers. I was terrified to discover that I knew more about this disease than the dermatologist did.

What I learned is there are no known causes, cures or answers about whether it will spread, turn into systemic scleroderma, or be inherited by the children I plan to have.

I am engaged to be married next fall and now I am not sure if I should still look forward to children and a normal life or if I am going to turn into a freak with patches all over my body before I get to take my wedding photos.

It has been six months since the first spot showed up and now it has grown to three distinct blotches in one spot and I am developing another on the back of my shoulder and one on my forearm both on the same side as the original spot.

Once I got home I found this Web site and began to read stories from other people with this disease. As sad as I am to hear these other horrible stories, it gives me some sort of hope that someday we may actually be able to put two and two together and find out some answers. I do not take the runaround easily, especially when it is about my body.

Several things that I have noticed as a common factor amongst stories are that many people with morphea seem to have had a lot of sun exposure before it first occurred. It seems no one has received the same treatments or answers from their doctors, and everyone seems to feel the same as I do.

I think there is a new emotion that develops when learning to deal with this disease. I am full of anger and frustration right now. Will someone please just give me some sort of answer I can grasp onto? I do not know what to believe, where to turn, what to try next, or what to tell people who care about me when they ask me questions.

I have noticed that sun exposure agitates the spots so I am learning to become nocturnal. I have also noticed that it only itches when the spots are very dry such as right after a shower, or after being in the sun, so I have been keeping lotion on it which helps with the itching.

My spots are pale white with darker rings on the outside of them. The skin is extremely shiny, tough, slick and scaly.

I wish with all my heart that every one of us would be writing in with our successful victory stories very soon. My heart goes out to each and every one of you suffering with the same disease.

Update – February 2004

It has been almost two years since my original diagnosis, so I am approaching the end of the time period where most cases disappear if they are going to disappear. I have been through the entire emotional roller coaster and I am feeling much more at peace with my disease. In fact, I try not to even look at it as a disease anymore.

I have found that the best way to deal with it is to keep living my life and not looking back. Since my diagnosis I have had several big events in my life.

Most importantly, I was married in September 2003, to my best friend who supports me through all the uncertainty. That has provided me with much happiness and a sense of balance in my life.

Also during this time I started to experience new ailments and I am still not certain if they pertain to this disease or from just plain stress. I started to feel a strange sensation in my esophagus, almost as if something were stuck inside. This sensation came and went, but sometimes it would stay for a few weeks at a time and then it would be gone. I underwent several tests which were not the least bit pleasant only to find out nothing.

A week later my heart began palpitating and causing me spurts of adrenaline and a dizzy sensation randomly throughout the day. I gave the symptoms one week in case it was the flu or a reaction to the barium they had me drink for a test the week prior. When it persisted I returned to the doctor. Once again they wanted to run more tests on me. I was reluctant, however, I felt my life was at stake and fear took over, so I finally agreed. They hooked me up to a twenty-four hour heart monitor. This found nothing wrong because the symptoms strangely disappeared that same day.

The symptoms did not show up again until almost exactly one year later when the same thing happened for one week and vanished. I was far less nervous the second time as I had already experienced the whole thing.

Currently I am experiencing nothing and I have written the esophagus problem off to heartburn. I am tired of being a guinea pig used by the doctors for speculation as a pawn to get insurance money for test after test. I am much happier when I stay away from the doctors and try to forget about the entire thing as much as possible. I try not to let it get me down.

During the winter it is far easier to deal with my morphea because it remains hidden. I somewhat dread the sunshine, but I have learned to deal with it as best as I can.

The spots have taken up my entire right arm, shoulder and are spreading across my back now. They do not show any signs of stopping, so I try not to get my hopes up anymore like I used to. It only leads to a greater let down each time it stays.

My biggest fear is one that I do not have much information on. My husband and I are dying to start a family. I am just afraid I either will not be able to have children, or if I am able, that they may end up with this same terrible disease. I would feel a huge amount of guilt if another person had to suffer with this disease because of me.

Editor's Note: There are some treatments for morphea now, however many cases do not need treatment. It is my understanding that morphea does not interfere with pregnancy, although some people need to discontinue certain medications for it, prior to attempting pregnancy. Please discuss this with your doctor or scleroderma expert.

Tami
Illinois, USA

I was diagnosed with morphea scleroderma when I was only five. I am now twenty-four and trying to lead what we call a normal life. Well, at least as normal as it can be, considering I have a disease that limits me from time to time.

I have fought being sick for as long as I can remember. I get tired very quickly if I do not slow down here and there. Right now I am battling severe muscle pain in my legs. My internist tells me it is not my scleroderma, but I still think it is probably related to it.

I have tried arthritis medications, muscle relaxers and water exercises. Nothing seems to help, and the pain comes and goes. Some days I feel like I could run a marathon and other days I can barely find the strength to get off the couch.

I work in the medical field and have come to the conclusion through all this there are always worse things in life and I can be thankful I can still stand tall most days, at least on the days that I find the strength to get off the couch.

I have gotten used to the stares everyone casts my way because in their eyes I am different. Unique, I guess. Where I am from there is no one around who has this disease that I am aware of. I am interested in talking with others and seeing how they cope day to day.

Update – October 2003

For the past six months I have been battling this disease and it seems like a year. I now suffer from narrowed patella-femoral joint spaces and am getting ready to start some injections for that. I hope that maybe they will give me a couple of good months.

I am twenty-five and find normal activities so strenuous now. There are times when I just want to throw in the towel and quit, but I keep telling myself there are worse things in life to suffer from, and I feel fortunate that I am able to still walk (or shall I say hobble) on my legs.

I think the only way I have been able to get through this so far has been because of my wonderful family. Without my mother by my side to support me I probably would not still be holding my chin up.

I just want everyone out there to know that we may feel like the world is caving in on us, but if we take a look around we can see that things could be worse.

Granted, I do look around from time to time and wish I did not have scleroderma, but I think God has a plan for all of us, even though I wonder what the plan involves for me.

I wish all of you the best and I hope you enjoy the good days!

Toni
New Zealand

I am in the process of discovering what scleroderma is all about. I was diagnosed as a child with a strange skin complaint, but was given no information about it. My mother does not remember what she was told either, so she has been of no help.

Then about two years ago I discovered more patches on my skin that seemed to be spreading. The skin specialist I saw gave it the name scleroderma or morphea. My treatment is cortisone cream applied twice daily, but I still do not know anything about the disease.

I am in my early forties. I have eight children and want to learn what I can about morphea. This is why I am sharing my story.

PART 3

Autoimmune and Overlap

CHAPTER 7

Autoimmune Stories

Then the rest of the pain wakes up
and my day begins.
—Jody

Danielle Lewis
Asthma
California, USA

In the year 2000, a bad winter hit Woodland Hills, California. I went to work via public transit to work night shift for my customer service job. I normally traveled thirty miles by bus, five and sometimes six days a week.

I bundled up the best I could. I had a cold and knew that I should not be out in the cold, but my employer was not sympathetic. Besides, I had been out sick for several days, and I needed the money.

Anyway, I was halfway through my shift when my coughing became uncontrollable, so I was sent home early, at three o'clock in the morning.

It was New Year's Eve, and the temperature was forty-two degrees Fahrenheit. The second bus had stopped running because of the holiday, so I walked to another bus stop, hoping that it would get me closer to home. As I walked, I felt my lungs wheezing, and my cough got even worse.

Then it began to rain. I knew that my cousin was asleep, but I had no choice but to call and wake her up. She rushed to pick me up, but by the time she had gotten to me, I was soaked and miserable.

The next day I went to the doctor and I was diagnosed with a bad case of bronchitis. I took medicine for it, and it got better. However, few weeks later I began to have the same symptoms, only this time I could not breathe at all, so my family rushed me to the emergency room.

The doctor said that I had an asthma attack. I was dumbfounded. I asked him if he was sure, since I have not had problems with my lungs, nor has anyone else in my family. As it turns out, I was diagnosed with Chronic Adult Onset Asthma.

After that, I got worse. I moved to Woodland Hills to be closer to my job, but I soon lost my job because of my frequent absences due to the illness. Because of the loss of my job, I acquired huge doctor and hospital bills. I could go to the county hospital, but the county emergency room is too far away when I have an asthma attack. So now I have emergency bills in almost all the hospitals near me, dating back almost two years.

I have tried desperately to find a job since then, and I have had to rethink my goals. I will have to work at home, because office environments are just too dusty and allergenic for me.

I wish I knew more about filing for disability for such an illness. I am not sure if asthmatics are even eligible for disability. Can I still file? Do I need to ask the county doctor if I can file for disability? What channels should I go through?

If I could manage a part-time job at home and also get disability, perhaps then I could get on the road to healing with my yoga breathing classes. And then I could also afford to move to another location with cleaner air.

Right now I am broke, with no bank account and no future. I am trying to develop some skills online and to get some work, but I have not found anything yet. Adapting to an asthmatic's lifestyle is the hardest thing that I have ever had to do

Faith Rumph
Eosinophilia-Myalgia Syndrome (EMS)
Virginia, USA

My name is Faith Rumph, and eosinophilia-myalgia syndrome (EMS) has altered my life forever. I am one of several thousand Americans who became ill from ingesting contaminated over-the-counter L-tryptophan, which is an amino acid dietary supplement. Many people were advised by their physicians in the 1980s to use tryptophan (L-T) for a variety of medical conditions, including chronic pain, premenstrual syndrome, and sleep disorders.

I used it for sleep and anxiety, but it did not help me very much with those difficulties. However, it rid me of the pain of occasional migraines and premenstrual syndrome, so I continued using the supplement.

Little did I know that the product was manufactured overseas, shipped in bulk to America, put into pill form and bottled here, and then sold under American companies' names, with no mention of the fact that the raw product originated in a foreign country. The bottles said tryptophan was pure, natural and safe. This is why I believe in labeling of dietary products so that consumers can know the country of origin, along with other information.

Then disaster struck.

On August 17, 1989, at age thirty-nine, I awoke with red, swollen, burning thighs. In all my life I had never seen anything like this painful, symmetrical rash. For two and a half years I would use L-T at the recommended dosage. To me, using L-T was like taking a vitamin supplement. It was a substance that I took and never imagined that it could cause real harm, or much less that it could cause a brand-new chronic disease.

Over the next few months I got worse, with one diagnosis after another, each becoming more serious as I saw one doctor after another. First, I was told I had hives. The medication for hives did nothing for my burning red legs. Soon the rash began to spread downward and upward, although it looked less ominous overall for a short time.

I was told I might have eczema; however a brilliant allergist actually said the following to me the first time he saw my legs: "I have never seen anything like this rash, and I do not know what it is." That was late August 1989. All these uncertainties took a terrible toll on my husband, and on my son, who was about twelve years old at the time.

In September, I worried I might be contracting rheumatoid arthritis when shooting electric-like pains coursed through my hands, wrists, legs, stomach, and even my head. As a highly trained pianist, I was terrified I would lose the use of my hands. I did not tell my doctors about these pains right away because I could not bear to hear that I might be getting a potentially crippling illness.

In October 1989, a dermatologist told me I had dermatitis, and advised me to look for things at home that might be causing the stinging, red rash that kept spreading and tormenting me relentlessly, with a hot, constant, burning pain.

I also had a small, white, scar-like spot on my right chest, and it began to grow bigger and thicker until it covered the whole right side of my chest and extended to the area near my armpit. At that point, I could not lift either arm normally.

Pain and I coexisted daily as I grew weaker. Rising from chairs and walking were hard for me to do without help. I coughed and had shortness of breath, but I attributed these things just to allergies.

Both of my legs became encrusted in a tough, thick yellowish-brown covering that prevented hair from growing, so I resembled a lizard. I lost about one-third of my scalp hair and all the fine hair on my body. My body hair eventually grew back, although only sparsely on my legs. My scalp hair has never regained its original fullness, either.

The most frightening symptom to me was the muscle spasms at night. Sometimes they occurred several times a night, starting in my feet and moving up my legs. They lasted for thirty to forty minutes and were accompanied by nausea, sweating, and an inability to move out of the bed. My feet felt as if they were caught in a bear trap, and it was the worst pain I have ever felt, except for natural childbirth.

In addition, my jaws often suddenly clamped shut when I was eating, and my teeth grew loose. Sometimes stomach spasms tore through my abdominal cavity, interfering with my breathing. At times it would feel like a hard ball was moving up my stomach to my rib cage; it would hold and then let go, and return to my lower abdomen. When the ball reached my rib cage, I felt as though I might suffocate.

All this time I continued to take tryptophan. I asked a doctor who diagnosed me in October with polymyositis if the tryptophan was okay to use. She answered, "This is so safe you could probably take one hundred pills at a time, and it would not do anything to you." So I continued to take the contaminated L-T.

Finally, in early November 1989, one of my doctors called and told me I had scleroderma, based on three biopsies he had recently done. He told me I would need to have every organ tested, and that scleroderma could be fatal. Just two weeks before he had still thought I only had dermatitis. I hung up the phone and cried. The next day I called a scleroderma organization.

A dizzying battery of tests began that went on until a few days before Christmas. I turned forty in late November. Every new day brought different symptoms and more generalized pain and weakness. I thought I was going to die, and I prepared to die.

However, on November 17th, we saw a newspaper article about a strange new disease. The disease had first been noted in New Mexico and had been connected to usage of tryptophan.

Eosinophilia and myalgia were symptoms of the new disease called eosinophilia-myalgia syndrome (EMS), and I had all the markers of it. I knew at once what was happening to me and stopped using L-T that day.

In my hopefulness, I believed the disease would go away completely in a month or two like an allergic reaction. Instead, the EMS worsened after I stopped using the pills. This was one of the cruelest aspects of EMS to me, that not using the pills did not stop the symptoms. In time, we all realized we had a novel disease and that we likely would always have it.

The Center For Disease Control and Prevention (CDC), National Institutes of Health (NIH), Food and Drug Administration (FDA), and Mayo Clinic all helped unravel the connection between tainted L-T and EMS. However, I do not think anyone at that time could have imagined that many of us with EMS would still be sick with the chronic phase of the disease. The many aspects of our puzzling illness often baffle our doctors.

I am lucky I have not had ascending paralysis or pulmonary hypertension, like some people. But I went on disability in 1997 and have the following problems among many others: tight skin on parts of my body (scleroderma-like skin); muscle weakness and pain; dry mouth and eyes; jaw and facial pain that is awful; inability to walk or stand for more than ten minutes at a time; and various diseases secondary to EMS, including fibromyalgia.

EMS is a multisystem, chronic, novel disease that affects the immune system and is caused by ingestion of contaminated L-T associated with a particular foreign manufacturer. It has ruined my hands so that I cannot play the music I spent a lifetime learning to perform.

I use a wheelchair in public much of the time, travel seldom and with hardship, only attend a few social engagements a year, and cannot get to church more than a few times annually.

But I am grateful to be alive, and I have immersed myself in the work of helping others with EMS. We need research funds, for instance. I recently launched a Web site, www.eosinophilia-myalgia.net, that offers information, support, and ideas for advocacy. I hope to see EMS included in some research projects of similar diseases, such as scleroderma, fibromyalgia, and Gulf War illnesses.

I do not want eosinophilia-myalgia syndrome to ever be forgotten or to ever happen again due to a similarly tainted product.

Jennifer Foster
Eosinophilic Fasciitis (EF)
Canada

I have eosinophilic fasciitis (EF). I am a twenty-seven year old English teacher living just north of Toronto, Ontario. In July 2000, I got married and on our honeymoon we went canoeing, biking, swimming and kayaking. I couldn't have felt better.

In November 2000, I started to have pain in my wrists and ankles. I had been rather lethargic and had gained some unwanted weight. I had started Tae Bo exercises, but I decided it was too hard on my joints, so I did a bit of cross-country skiing in December instead.

I complained to my doctor of pain and tightness in my arms, and he said that was a common thing for cross country skiers. By Christmas I could not get up comfortably from a seated position on the floor.

I see now I was in major denial. By February I had extreme swelling, pitted edema, and joint contractures in my knees and wrists. I could not make a fist or straighten my hand.

I had started a routine of only work and sleep. I ached with every step I took, and when I stretched, I felt rockets of pain and a sensation of prolonged and painful flexing of the muscles even after the movement had stopped. I could not open a water bottle. I also could not turn the ignition key, let alone belt myself into the car.

I am happy to report that my complaints at this time were heeded by doctors and due to their expertise my improvement has been phenomenal. When my family doctor saw my swollen limbs, he sent me to an internist who noted I have heart problems. My tricuspid valve was moderately regurgitating.

He put me on a diuretic, and I lost fifteen pounds of water weight in two weeks. I normally weigh one hundred and twelve pounds so that was a lot of weight loss. They thought this edema was due to my heart irregularities, but I know now that it was the first sign of this disease. Since the cardiology concerns were also new, I think the tissue disorder triggered the tricuspid insufficiency.

I met with a cardiologist in Toronto who ordered a transesophageal echocardiogram since I had already had a regular echocardiogram. But he could not explain the stiffness and hardness in my limbs.

He sent me to a rheumatologist, who said the problem was dermatological. I had developed very limited movement. I had a pigmented and hardened line on my forearm and shiny irregular skin along my shins.

I taught school every day, which luckily was in a school with no stairs. At night I came home to sleep on the couch, before climbing upstairs on my fists. I could no longer open my hands, so I had developed very interesting penmanship.

In April I was prescribed prednisone. I have heard nightmare tales about it, but prednisone became my saving grace, despite some nasty cosmetic side effects.

Dermatology saw me for 'rounds' and that is where I first heard of eosinophilic fasciitis (EF). I had developed a white shiny patch of skin on my back. I had skin biopsies taken on my forearm and on my back. The results for my arm were inconclusive since the biopsy was not deep enough. The second and deeper biopsy was taken after I had already been administered large doses of prednisone.

My eosinophils in the blood samples were eleven percent. The patch on my back was identified as generalized morphea. It has not grown.

In June I was feeling better due to prednisone and diuretics. My feet were painful and I could not point my toes, but I actually wore heels to a wedding!

I started to call myself "Puff Jenny" due to a fat face. As a young teacher I have to face teenagers every day, and I was feeling embarrassed by my moon face and dark facial hair. However, being able to climb stairs without much pain and only minimal awkwardness nicely combats my vanity.

I stopped the diuretics in the summer as I was dehydrated and I did not seem to have swelling anymore. I am tapering off the prednisone, and I have just ended a year of physiotherapy with ultrasound. I am feeling hopeful and nearly normal.

My husband has been extraordinarily accepting of the rapid deterioration of my once charming and petite figure. I have gained about eighteen pounds from the prednisone. My back and stomach are fatty, and because of my puffy face I jokingly say, "I am storing nuts for the winter." But hey, I can make a fist now. Wish me luck!

◆ ❖ ◆

Susan
Eosinophilic Fasciitis (EF)
Texas, USA

I was diagnosed with eosinophilic fasciitis (EF) in June 1999. It is a scleroderma-like illness, which is also known as Shulman's Syndrome. My kidneys had just failed after having glomerulonephritis for over thirty years.

While I was in the hospital and starting dialysis, my right arm became swollen and hard as a rock. After going to dialysis for about three months, I kept getting worse. My whole body turned to wood. I could hardly move. I thought it was caused by dialysis.

One day I told my doctor that if he could not find out what was wrong with me soon, I would not be here very much longer. I was ready to end it all, because losing my kidneys and having a body like wood was getting to be just too much for me.

My doctor did some research and sent me to the Texas Medical Center to see a rheumatologist. The rheumatologist knew what I had right away, since he had two other patients with the same thing. He took a deep tissue biopsy, which confirmed my illness. He started me on medications, and in a short time the hardness went away. I have had EF for three years now.

In August 2001, I had a kidney transplant. My new kidney is doing great, however, I am now fighting myopathy from cholesterol medications. They tell you to notify your doctor if you develop muscle weakness from cholesterol medication, and I did, but my doctors ignored me.

After three months I quit the medicine on my own, because I just knew deep down that the medicine was causing this. Also, my rheumatologist ordered a test of my muscles, and that is what they found. I have been in pain from the myopathy for five months. It is gradually getting better, but I have a long way to go.

When I first got EF, my symptoms were itchy skin at night, and skin hardness. I could not wash my hair or bathe myself, since I could not raise my arms. I could not cook, clean or even get out of a chair without help. Once, I tried to make a sandwich and it took me forty-five minutes, as I had to rest after each step. My hands were also very weak and I could not open jars.

Because of the skin hardness, I could not be put on the kidney transplant list. Also I could not have a graft put under my skin. I had a catheter in my chest for eighteen months.

Finally I was able to get the graft and then get put on the transplant list. It took me eleven months to get a kidney. When I did, I was the only match for this kidney in the whole United States!

Right before my transplant, I was feeling pretty good. The EF was only affecting my skin. I was swimming laps and even played a little racquetball. I bet I would be doing that now, if it were not for the muscle problem.

I was lucky, as medications have been successful in helping my disease. There were days when I was depressed, but now I keep going and know there must be a reason to have this, and I hope my story will help others.

Jody
Fibromyalgia and Difficult Diagnosis
Florida, USA

Each day begins the same. Before I even open my eyes, I feel the pain in my hands. I swallow and feel the pain in my throat. Then the rest of the pain wakes up and my day begins. I feel like I am drowning in a sea of ambiguity.

I was in the midst of an around-the-world expedition when I fell ill. I had difficulty acclimating to the heat and preferred air conditioning. In Kenya, I was bitten by an unknown insect and my hand and arm swelled up. In Sudan, I was on intravenous fluids for heat stroke and food poisoning. And in Thailand, at the end of March, it all came to a crashing halt.

I was in a scuba diving course and I became very cold in the water. My instructor said she had Raynaud's, explained what it was, and offered me a spare wet suit.

The wet suit helped a lot, but a few days later, I presented with signs of decompression sickness. After three days I was treated with a total of ten hours in a hyperbaric chamber, but afterwards I still had symptoms, including blurred vision, tingling in my hands and feet, and vertigo.

I was going to fly to Bangkok to see another doctor. The day I was to head out, I developed red blotches and tiny blisters on my hands.

In Bangkok I saw many doctors at a top-notch hospital. I couldn't see clearly out of my glasses and three opticians were unable to help. I saw the hospital ophthalmologist, who, without dilating my eyes, said I had swollen optic nerves.

He said, "You need a CAT scan. Something is wrong in your brain." I attributed his tactless approach to English not being his native language. My CAT scan came back normal. MRIs showed bulges to the disks in my neck, and the doctor thought this explained my vertigo.

The dermatologist said my hand symptoms were due to urticarial vasculitis. All labs came back normal except one; my antinuclear antibody (ANA) was positive at 1:320 with a speckled pattern. No explanation was given to me as to what this meant.

I was released from the hospital and put in physical therapy. I kept my room air conditioner on at sixty-two degrees and was comfortable. I discontinued physical therapy because of pain. I saw another doctor several days later and she redid my MRIs, with contrast. At this point my neck and shoulder blades felt desensitized. My vertigo was worsening.

The MRIs showed inflammation to my cervical spine, the nerves and nerve roots, and four cranial nerves. The doctor said it was post-infectious immune mediated with no further explanation except that doctors in the United States did not know what this was, but she could treat it there.

I was given a three day treatment, with no information about the side effects. I was also given medication for fibromyalgia. The doctor said not to worry, that I did not have lupus or multiple sclerosis, and I would be fine.

When I got home, I eventually saw a neurologist. He thought I had a connective tissue disease, maybe vasculitis, and that I needed a work up done. I did not have health insurance, and could not afford these tests. I was feeling better and stopped taking my medicine, as I thought I would be fine. He suggested I could be seen at a free clinic where he volunteered.

At the free clinic, on June 28th, one day after the general practitioner suggested I had Behcet's disease, but was in remission, I started to relapse. I felt like I had arthritis in my hip and hands. My neck was going numb and it was hard to breathe deeply. I looked up Behcet's, but it did not really fit with my symptoms.

I spent the fourth of July in the emergency room. My erythrocyte sedimentation rate (ESR) was seventeen and I was admitted for chest pain. The next day another neurologist saw me and said I needed a full work-up and that he thought I had lupus or a connective tissue disease. I had to leave the hospital as I was paying out of pocket and could not afford to stay or have any more tests done.

I spent the next week sleeping, hardly eating, and feeling lousy. What energy I had was used on the computer reading up on everything I could. I thought I had thoracic outlet syndrome. I made an appointment to be seen by a local doctor who specialized in problems related to diving, as I thought that perhaps my symptoms were due to residual decompression sickness. Maybe it was a fibromyalgia response to so much prednisone, or to going cold turkey off my medicines.

I noticed that my right hand would always get cold when I was on the computer and I figured it was from resting on my wrist when I used the mouse. I read up on lupus, MS and vasculitis. With each minute that passed I would become entrenched in fear.

I then went to the county hospital to get into their rheumatology clinic. My ESR was 5. My ANA was 1:160 homogenous and speckled. The doctors there did not seem to listen to my complaints and said I had no clinical signs of lupus or any connective tissue disease, that I just had fibromyalgia.

The dive doctor said, "You do not go diving and come out with lupus." He did not want to treat me until he knew of the results of follow up tests.

In August both of my hands were getting cold when I typed. I had a sore throat that no one checked, and I was fatigued. I went to a chiropractor who did some adjustments. I stopped going when she adjusted my neck and left me with a nonstop pulsating sensation that went from the back of my neck into my head. It felt like the arteries were pounding like a fast-paced heartbeat that faded and then came back. Now it feels like a tugging sensation. My scalp gets sore and my eyes bother me.

I saw an infectious disease doctor who said it all seemed post infectious and that depending on new MRI results, I might need a spinal tap.

Then I went to a neuro-opthamologist who said he saw nothing wrong neurologically that could explain my new symptoms. I saw stars and floaters when I was outside. I told him I went to the optician because I had blood shot eyes for about a week and he tried to dilate my eyes but they would not dilate with the initial drops he used. He had to use other drops. My eyes stayed dilated for two days after seeing the neuro-opthamologist. He said it seemed fibromyalgia related, and that I needed a pain management program and physical therapy. He also said he thought my MRIs were over-read in Thailand and did not agree with the cranial neuritis diagnosis.

The MRI result appeared stable in comparison to previous ones. It showed maybe some increased signals in my spine and a vascular anomaly that had been there previously. The doctor did not find neuritis in certain nerves in my head. Basically the doctor thought my MRI seemed fine. The neurologist said the pulsation could be due to irritation to the tiny nerves in my neck that cannot be seen in an MRI.

But my hands were still annoying me. They would become speckled red all the time. They were generally cold, especially when I typed. My feet seemed cold too, but they have always been that way. In the mornings, my hands hurt and felt rubbery when water touched them. I was taking several baths a day to alleviate muscle pain and the pulsation in my neck, and I felt I had dishpan hands.

I was getting reflux at night and my hips really hurt. I was in physical therapy and could not handle the water class. The water, though it was ninety degrees, bothered my hands and they would prune easily. I was getting tiny blisters on my fingers and thought it was Raynaud's. My wrists hurt too much to do the exercises.

I started to wake up with numb hands and I panicked. Then I read up on carpal tunnel syndrome and this seemed logical since I was on the computer so much. I was told by a few doctors that my symptoms could all be stemming from my neck and shoulders.

The doctor who specialized in divers said he wanted to treat me and thought this arthritis pain I had was residual decompression sickness. The diving insurance company from Australia declined coverage since I had been repatriated, which is an exclusion clause I was never privy to and that I still contest with them.

I have since been back to the neurologist, who disregards my cold red hands and says my problems are rheumatological and he thinks I have vasculitis.

My best friend was visiting from New York for two weeks in October. I had been waiting months for this visit and was very disappointed to be so fatigued. One day I took an anti-inflammatory for a headache and we headed out for a day at South Beach. We had sushi for lunch and my stomach began to bother me.

When I got home and went to the bathroom, I passed some blood. I spent five hours in the emergency room and was admitted with pancreatitis. There was no explanation as to what caused it other than perhaps the non-steroidal anti-inflammatory pills. I told the emergency room doctor it hurt when I ate. He asked how long it had felt this way and I said since June.

I argued with the attending doctor to check my ESR to see if it was high. I told the gastroenterology doctor that I had a sore throat and reflux, but no one checked my throat. I had a sigmoidoscopy done. I had had one last year before I left on my trip because I have irritable bowel syndrome (IBS). They found internal hemorrhoids, ergo the blood. After two days on IV and liquids only, my enzymes went down, my ESR was 6, and I was released.

Three days later, after attending a wedding and going snorkeling, I had a terrible sore throat and my voice was shot. I spent seven hours waiting to see a doctor at an urgent care clinic and she said she thought it was from my postnasal drip and reflux. I sleep on my back because my shoulders bother me. She said to sleep propped up against pillows. She gave me reflux medication and it helped almost immediately.

Yesterday I went back to the rheumatologist. I wanted to discuss my symptoms and how I felt that no one was listening and that I was afraid the doctors are missing something. Last week I discovered this Web site and started to panic seeing my symptoms in one arena. I would not question my having fibromyalgia if I wasn't ANA positive. With that, though, anything goes.

My parents took off work to go to the doctor with me. A general practitioner saw me because the rheumatologist was busy with other patients. So there I was with another doctor who had no specialty in rheumatology. Every doctor I have seen seems to pass the buck to the next and I cannot even discuss my symptoms with the doctor I want. On this visit I was in tears as soon as the doctor asked how I was. But he seemed genuinely concerned and told me to start from the beginning.

Slowly I explained my symptoms and that I have symptoms that are going untreated. I showed him the page I printed off the web with CREST signs. I said I have reflux and I have Raynaud's. My parents interjected that I sit in the house with a sweatshirt on. I said I have little spider veins on my face that I never noticed before. At the same time I developed Raynaud's I was waking up with numb hands and thought I had carpal tunnel syndrome.

I told him the neurologist would not do anything right now because I am seeing a top neurologist in December, and he wants to wait and see what that doctor says. He listened and listened and I decided I wanted him to be my general practitioner, since I did not really have one.

The rheumatologist came in and said she understood my concerns but right now there was no clinical suggestion of scleroderma. The SCL-70 test was negative. She said my ANA does not have an anti-centromere pattern. I told her that SCL-70 is not positive in everyone, and I do have symptoms. I guess it does not matter that my symptoms appeared even more strongly after the labs were drawn in July.

The rheumatologist said she knows it was frustrating with people in the beginning, because the symptoms I have can appear in all connective tissue diseases, and they have to monitor it to see if it progresses.

They set up EMG tests for carpal tunnel and gastrointestinal tests for reflux. Again, since it is a public health system and they are overwhelmed with other uninsured people, the tests are not going to be done until next March.

The doctor said, "You have been doing plenty of research and you know there is no treatment or cure for scleroderma, and it isn't like you want a diagnosis." I would not be able to get insurance and it would not change my symptoms or my pain.

She said I had significant fibromyalgia, which has all the symptoms I have been experiencing, and that it is her job to monitor me and follow the progression. She said what I really need is proper sleep and suggested I try a medication to help me sleep.

I cannot get work. I cannot get health insurance. I cannot seem to get better. The only thing I can seem to get is upset. Each night I go to sleep and think that tomorrow I will be back to normal.

Update – April 2003

My ANA is negative. I have gastroparesis and mild reflux/dysmotility that occurs with gastroparesis. My peristalsis is normal, but the waves of peristalsis are uncoordinated and sometimes go into spasm, especially if I drink something hot or cold.

My doctors insist this isn't scleroderma, but rather is idiopathic. My manometry yielded nonspecific symptoms with no known etiology to explain it. My fingers still get cold when I use the computer, and my fingertips generally get pinkish or red. They do not turn white or blue, they just get ruddy and the doctors say that it is not typical Raynaud's.

They are not sure if it is brought on by thoracic outlet syndrome or neck problems or what. These symptoms annoy me most. It happens every day, several times a day including whenever I type, which is a tough problem for a writer. I can change the color of my hands and temperature just by moving my neck and shoulders around.

I will see a neurologist in a few weeks. I have ulnar problems but the carpal tunnel test was fine. They never tested my neck though, and all my problems stem from my neck and shoulders.

I am a lot better than I was a year ago. I still have the gnawing fear that this is all related, turning into something terrible and my doctors just don't know any better. But there is not anything that can reverse findings in modern medicine, especially when my blood work comes back normal.

The fear does not consume me as it once did, perhaps because I am occupying my time doing things other than researching symptoms. I am trying a lot of alternative treatments. I use my treadmill almost every day or do yoga. And I am searching for a job.

Update —May 2003

My ANA came back positive again, at 1:160 mixed. My rheumatologist still claims that she thinks I am a false positive.

I am in San Francisco and undergoing a series of hyperbaric oxygen treatments to try to curb whatever is happening to me. I am constantly chilled. My fingers have become icy and bother me whenever I am not in direct sunlight. If I touch something in the refrigerator, they drain of color momentarily and then take on the same appearance as they always have with the fingertips a little pink and the temperature cold, or the color is completely normal but they are still icy, as well as my nose and toes, too.

I am sick of being sick. I am sick of worrying. And I am sick of doctors who either know nothing, or who just do not want to deal with this. I resent the fact that I am forced to spend so much time researching information, scaring myself while I am at it. I am told I should have more faith in my doctors, that I need to let the doctors do their job, but how in the world can I?

I just have to hold out hope that the hyperbaric treatments will work and regulate my immune system. If we don't have hope, what do we have?

◆ ❖ ◆

Keri
Undiagnosed
Canada

I am a thirty-one years old, and I have been living with back pain, stomach problems and skin problems since I was a teenager.

After seeing many specialists, I have a diagnosis for my spinal pain that has left me with no treatment and no answers. They have diagnosed me with a herniated disc in my lower back, which is causing me a lot of pain, and Scheuermann's Disease (curvature of the spine) in my upper back, which also causes me pain.

I have continual stomach problems. Somtimes my heart palpitates like it is jumping out of my chest. I have had anemia for three years and have seen a specialist, but still have no answers.

I have had acne all my life and recently saw a skin specialist who diagnosed me with acne rosacea and dermatitis, with eczema.

Some days my pain is intolerable. I have headaches and fatigue almost every day. Most mornings I wake up feeling like I have a hangover. My mouth and lips are dry. I am tired all day and my stomach feels bloated.

◆ ❖ ◆

Sherrell
Undiagnosed
Arizona, USA

I am a forty-seven years old. I have been diagnosed with carpal tunnel syndrome (CTS) in my right elbow. I was sent to an orthopedic surgeon for a consultation. When he examined me, he mentioned that I may have scleroderma. He said my fingers and face showed signs of this disease.

I have visited some Web sites and found that I have some of the symptoms. I have irritable bowel syndrome (IBS) and daily heartburn. I also had to have a full set of dentures when I was twenty-nine years old. I am a chronic asthmatic and have stridor.

I have an appointment with my doctor to have further tests done to see if I have scleroderma. I take prednisone when my asthma acts up, but that always weakens my immune system. Hopefully, I will have further news after I see the doctor.

CHAPTER 8

Overlap, UCTD and MCTD Stories

I divide my life into two different time periods:
before I got sick, and after.

—Monica

Dotty
California, USA

I have just started chemotherapy with the first of six monthly infusion treatments that will hopefully control my very aggressive scleroderma condition that was diagnosed in June 2001.

My involvement with autoimmune disease started in the spring of 1998. One morning, I bit into a fresh orange and nearly went through the ceiling in pain. My body shook for about twenty seconds and it felt as if someone stabbed me with a knife in the temple near my ear.

For the next sixteen hours, I could not even take a teaspoon of water. My parotid gland bulged out like a golf ball. The next morning things were pretty normal. I had no pain and I could eat anything. The gland was down to a slight swelling. I went to see my doctor. She confirmed it was the parotid gland and told me if it happened again to come right in without an appointment so she could see it.

The next attack was three weeks later on a Saturday evening. By Monday morning, things were normal again except for a swollen parotid gland. Within six weeks I had three attacks and was referred to an ear, nose and throat (ENT) doctor, who found I had calcified particles, or stones, in my parotid gland. The lining of the gland duct was very thin in several places, indicating damage. My blood test showed very high levels of antinuclear antibodies (ANA).

My doctor explained the dangers of surgery that included possible damage to the nerves in the surgical area. I knew I could not sit around and wait for another attack. I was afraid to eat, never knowing when I would get another flare.

Since I decided to have surgery, my doctor did not take a lip biopsy to confirm Sjögren's syndrome, as the parotid gland would be biopsied. The tissue was sent to the University of Pittsburgh Medical Center for diagnosis (I live in California.) The results were startling. Not only did it confirm that I have Sjögren's but I am one of the four percent of Sjögren's patients with parotid lymphoma (Zone B cell, Malt type). After a total body CAT scan, they also found that I had lymphoma of the nasal pharynx.

My radiation oncologist was optimistic about the results of treatment. I had six weeks of head and neck radiation five times a week. Two weeks after starting treatment, my entire mouth blistered up. I could not eat or sip anything because of the pain. I was treated with an anesthetic mixture which numbed my mouth so I could have liquids. Food was out of the question. For a month I lived on supplemental nutrient drinks. There were times when the pain was so severe, I would put a tablespoon of the anesthetic mixture in my mouth and keep it there for two to three hours.

Other than my mouth and extreme fatigue, I was fine. The important thing is that I went into total remission. It has been more than three years since I completed radiation and I am doing fine. Surgery was one hundred percent successful. But after radiation, I completely lost my taste buds. Bananas were salty, and all food tasted bitter to me.

Although I was on a drug to help create moisture in mouth and eyes, I still had a very dry mouth and needed fluid to help get the miserable food down. I could not tolerate any kind of fruit or vegetables, whether raw, steamed or canned. I continued to depend on two cans of supplemental nutrient drinks daily and I tried different foods to find anything tolerable.

When a new drug appeared for treating dry mouth, I changed to it and six weeks later my taste buds returned to almost normal. I still cannot eat raw fruits and vegetables, although steaming helps.

I was fine until January 2001, when I diagnosed myself with Raynaud's phenomenon. I also found that I could not talk when I walked up a flight of stairs. I reported this to my doctor when I had my annual physical checkup in May. She looked at my fingers near my nails and said I had scleroderma. I could see nothing and thought she was nuts. I went home quite hysterical as I knew one person with a very severe case of scleroderma. After studying about it on the Internet, I realized that everyone was different and I must take hold of my emotions and do what has to be done.

A chest X ray confirmed mild pulmonary fibrosis, so I was referred to a pulmonologist and rheumatologist. In July 2001, a pulmonary function test (PFT) indicated a fifty percent rate of diffusion, which the doctor considered mild. My blood test was negative. He said he must treat the symptoms and ignore the blood test. He said my illness was mild and I would do fine.

In October I caught a slight cold and developed acute bronchitis. My lungs cleared up in two to three weeks after treatment, however, I still had a terrible cough. Sometimes I could not stop coughing for two to three hours. I was fine when I laid down, but the it would start again as soon as I sat or stood up.

My doctor said I had severe trauma to my system and it could take three to four months to clear up. It made sense, but I was very sick all winter.

I noticed a warning on one of my new medicines which said to be careful about taking it if you have pulmonary problems. I took myself off the drug, and within forty-eight hours my coughing stopped. I assume this drug was causing a buildup of mucus in my lungs. My mouth is much drier now, but at least I do not cough.

Prior to getting bronchitis, I had been swimming a half mile three times a week and working out with three pound weights. Within a short time, I could barely walk twenty-five feet without being short of breath.

In February 2002, I attended a Sjögren's Syndrome Foundation support meeting in San Diego. Dr. Robert Fox, a nationally recognized rheumatologist and an authority on Sjögren's, was the guest speaker. I had the opportunity to speak to him about my problem and he was most gracious to me. He told me I must have a high-resolution chest CAT scan to see what is really going on in the lungs and an echocardiogram to see if I have pulmonary hypertension (PH).

The results were good and bad. I did not have pulmonary hypertension, but my lungs were much worse. The fibrosis was very advanced, with only thirty percent diffusion. In approximately eight months, I went down from fifty percent to thirty-three percent. This should have taken many years, rather than months.

In addition, all the lymph nodes in my chest were double the size as compared to the scan taken in 1998. Naturally lymphoma was suspected, since I had history of the condition. I had a mediastinoscopy, which is surgery that allows the doctor to view middle of the chest and remove lymph nodes between the lungs to test them for cancer or infection. Every lymph node visible to the surgeon was removed and biopsied. Good news: no lymphoma! It was the scleroderma that had enlarged the nodes.

During these months my hands swelled and turned red and my skin thickened. I could feel my face tightening, and red spots began to appear. I was also losing my hair. I developed microstomia (small mouth) and bits of food started getting caught in my throat. My gastroesophageal reflux disease (GERD), worsened, along with my fatigue.

I have controlled my dental problems by being very conscious of dental care. I do not eat unless I can brush my teeth afterwards. I give my teeth a fluoride treatment daily. I floss twice a day, which is difficult because of my small mouth. My husband claims I will wear out my teeth, but my dentist says I am doing great.

My rheumatologist knew how he wanted to treat me, but he discussed the situation with Dr. Robert Fox and my original oncologist. They both agreed with him on taking very aggressive steps. I am receiving intravenous chemotherapy once a month for six months.

Once again I did my homework on the Internet and I found wonderful reports on this treatment. I found a 1998 report by researchers at John Hopkins Oncology Center on treating autoimmune disorders with chemotherapy.

The results were very exciting. The report talked about remission or at least partial remission by reprogramming the immune system with this treatment I know mental attitude is eighty percent of the battle. After seeing these reports, I find myself on cloud nine and looking forward to six months of treatment, hopefully going into some sort of remission, and getting a new lease on life.

My thoughts went to the latest medical technology. I told myself if modern research will help me, the least I can do is try to also help myself. Where one month ago I could not walk twenty-five feet, I am now walking one mile every day in thirty minutes. I have a lot to be thankful for. I may have been through a lot these last few years, but I have also been very lucky. It could have been much worse. I am not currently in pain. I am not in a wheelchair. I am not bedridden.

My husband and I celebrated our fiftieth wedding anniversary a month before I got bronchitis. I was in wonderful health for the party and enjoyed it thoroughly.

I am very upbeat about the chemotherapy I have just started getting. I just know it will help. I have taken control of my life and I know there is a wonderful future for me.

◆❖◆

Heidi M. Nolan
Nebraska, USA

I am forty years old and was diagnosed with undifferentiated connective tissue disease (UCTD) about one year ago.

Approximately two years ago I started noticing that my hands would go numb at night. I mentioned this problem to my general practitioner during an annual checkup. She thought that I had carpal tunnel syndrome (CTS) and sent me to a neurologist for an electrical conduction test. The neurologist said it was doubtful I had carpal tunnel, maybe borderline in my right hand, but my left hand was normal. Both hands went equally numb at night. The neurologist asked whether or not my doctor had checked me for Raynaud's or lupus.

I got on the Internet and started reading about Raynaud's and lupus. Although my hands are always cold, I had not yet noticed any color changes. However, when I read some of the symptoms of lupus, I wondered if I might have it because I had fatigue, oral ulcers, and frequent bouts of dizziness and headaches.

I called my general practitioner and asked to be tested for lupus. I did have elevated antinuclear antibodies (ANA), but that the specific test for lupus was negative. Since the results suggested some type of autoimmune disorder, she referred me to a rheumatologist.

When I saw the rheumatologist, he noticed my puffy fingers and thought it was odd that I did not have more wrinkles on my forehead. Nevertheless, he did not tell me anything was wrong. He just asked me to come back in six months to see how things progressed.

The next six months were unremarkable except for two things. I developed pinpoint-size sores on the tips of my fingers, which lasted about a month. I also noticed small areas of skin hardening at the base of both index fingers. My hands also felt burnt and itchy, as if I had been clapping for a long time.

When I saw the rheumatologist in November 2001, he diagnosed me with undifferentiated connective tissue disease (UCTD) and said that I might be developing scleroderma. He offered to put me on an antirheumatic medication, but I declined it because I was not having any symptoms that were interfering with my daily functioning.

During the end of November, I began having daily heartburn. In December I had diarrhea for twenty days. I also began to regurgitate my meals. I do not know if what I am calling regurgitation is what others refer to as acid reflux, but shortly after eating lunch and dinner, I would begin to burp and my mouth would fill with undigested food, which I would then have to spit out.

This would last anywhere from one to four hours after eating the meal and ranged from one to thirty ounces at a time. Also, my scalp became extremely itchy and I developed small open sores all over my chest.

The gastroenterologist did an endoscopy and a colonoscopy, and dilated my esophagus. He did not find any physical evidence of scleroderma, and the biopsies were normal. He started me on a drug for heartburn and regurgitation, but it did nothing for me.

Then he did a twenty-four-hour esophageal PH monitoring test, an esophageal manometry test, and a gastric emptying test. The PH test indicated I was having frequent reflux that was reaching my upper esophagus, but each reflux was brief (because when it came up, I spit it out.)

The esophageal manometry indicated some nonspecific dysmotility. Out of the ten swallows, two were a bit abnormal, but not enough to explain my regurgitation. The gastric emptying test was normal.

I was having horrible daily headaches that I thought were a side effect of the heartburn medication, so he started me on another one, but again, with no effect.

Throughout the winter months, my hands had begun to turn blue, purple and white when they were very cold, and bright red from getting hot when I was washing dishes

I saw the rheumatologist again in May and because there was no physical evidence of scleroderma, my diagnosis remained UCTD. He was not able to explain the physiological mechanism responsible for my regurgitation problems, but he thought it might represent a dysmotility problem. He started me on a pain medication for my headaches.

By August, the sores on my chest were gone and the regurgitation had completely stopped. Since the medicine I was taking never seemed to make a difference, I stopped taking all of it. Within a week, I was so stiff and sore from joint pain in my knees, wrists, and lower back, that I started the pain medication again.

Now it is mid-October and I think everything is starting back up. My fingertips are very tender, but I have not noticed any sores. I wake up two to four times every night with my hands in agony. They feel stiff, swollen, burning and numb. I find I have to put them on something cool and wiggle my fingers around a lot to help them feel better.

When I first get up, it is painful to put any weight on my feet. My soles feel very sensitive and my toes are sore. As the day progresses, my hands and feet feel much better.

In general, I can tell the quality of the skin on my hands is changing. It just feels thicker and kind of waxy. My forehead is very itchy and feels rougher than the rest of my face. The skin on my face in general is much pinker than it used to be.

My hands are frequently cold and I have noticed that they are blue and purple more often. I have also regurgitated my dinner three times in the last week.

I am thankful for the loving support of my adoring husband and my family. I know without a doubt that they will stand by and support me no matter what direction the disease may take.

Laura M.
New York, USA

I am forty-three, and after ten years of symptoms, tests, and doctor visits, I have been diagnosed with undifferentiated connective tissue disease (UCTD).

I have extreme fatigue, which keeps me in bed for days at a time. I also have muscle weakness, Raynaud's, extreme nausea, abdominal pain, joint pain, temperomandibular joint (TMJ) pain, low tone hearing loss in both ears, hair loss, lots of upper respiratory infections, slow wound healing, and the list goes on. I have finally had to quit my job, which I loved, but I have been out sick for too many days and each time I go back to work the cycle of sick days and good days starts again.

The rheumatologists that I have seen have done the following for me: Told me to stop wasting my life, that I am not sick. Patted me on the knee and told me to come back in two months. Diagnosed me with lupus and put me on antirheumatic medication which made my symptoms worse. Told me I did not look sick and to "get a life."

As anyone who is going through this knows, having the doctors treat us this way just causes more stress. I had found a wonderful immunologist who diagnosed me with UCTD and referred me to yet another rheumatologist, who again told me to stop wasting my life trying to find out what is wrong. This was after I told her that I had been out sick fifty-six workdays over the past year and have finally had to quit my job. Her response was that I was probably depressed and that the depression would get worse with quitting my job. She prescribed an antidepressant. This was after telling me I did not have an illness! Ugh.

If anyone reads this and is going through the same problems, I would love to hear from you. People who are not feeling these symptoms have a difficult time understanding. I cannot tell you how many people tell me I do not look sick after they ask how I am feeling. And then, of course, they come up with their own reasons why I feel like this.

I hope this helps someone else see that they are not alone, because sometimes it feels like that to me.

❖❖❖

Lynn
Indiana, USA

It will be a year in July since I got my diagnosis. I went to a specialist because of loss of hearing in my right ear. He put me through many tests and also an MRI, thinking it could be a tumor. The test came back negative. He was unable to find the problem.

In the meantime I was in my home walking around when suddenly my leg locked up at the hip and pelvic. The pain was so bad I could hardly stand it. The next day I went to the emergency room. The doctor took X rays and said it must be a pulled muscle and sent me home with muscle relaxers, which did not help a bit.

I went to see my family doctor, but she had just taken pregnancy leave, so I saw a nurse practitioner, which I would not have done under normal conditions, but my pain was awful and it was not getting any better. She seemed concerned and sent me to the hospital for a CT scan.

They could not give me the dye because of my veins collapsing, so they said if there were any problems they should show up, but maybe not as clear as they could be. The scan came back normal, and my nurse practitioner said my problem could be constipation, and she told me to take laxatives. Needless to say, that was the end of my visits to the nurse practitioner.

I then went to see my husband's doctor, who was a specialist in bone and sports medicine. He took X rays, but nothing showed up. I was beginning to think I was nuts.

He told me that sometimes hairline cracks did not always show up. He sent me to the hospital for a full body scan. The test showed I had a fractured pelvis. He said, "You need to see your family physician, because to fracture for no reason is unusual." This had happened in September and here it was January. I was still limping and thought I would never be able to walk normally again.

Then after I had given up on my hearing, the ear specialist called me and said that I needed to come in to discuss my abnormal blood work. I was nervous when it was put to me in such a matter of fact way. This blood work had been taken in July and here it was January. I did not understand why it had taken so long. It turned out that I had been so distracted with my pelvic problem that I had forgotten about my ear and had missed some of my ear specialist appointments.

The doctor asked, "Have you been feeling okay and where have you been?" Then he told me I had lupus, scleroderma, Sjogren's, and polymyositis overlap. He made me an appointment with a rheumatologist. Since then I still have no hearing in my right ear and my hands have been affected. I have a hard time opening lids and I also have to be careful to not skin my fingers, as they heal very slowly.

I am going to start to see the doctor more often and take better care of myself. I think I am somewhat still in denial but I know now that it is not just symptoms I have, but a disease. I hope my story helps someone who is also looking for answers.

Monica
Pennsylvania, USA

I am a thirty-four year old wife and mother of four. I divide my life into two different time periods: before I got sick, and after.

My life has never been normal. I had Reye's syndrome, which caused liver failure and brain swelling, at age eight. I spent two weeks in the hospital, including one week in a coma. There were eight other children who were brought in with the same symptoms, but I was the only one to survive. I was the lucky one to have gotten the fresh-out-of-medical-school resident at the time of entering the emergency room. I survived that time with no lasting problems.

When I was twenty-seven, I started having blackouts, migraines, and being just plain tired. My doctor started treating the symptoms as they appeared. There never seemed to be a great deal of alarm until I started having seizure-like activity. My mother's mother-in-law died of epilepsy but I brushed off the test that would later show positive for a seizure disorder.

In the fall of 1997, I suffered a grand mal seizure that lasted twenty-five minutes and almost claimed my life. My husband walked in on this and turned me over just in time. I knew then I needed to seek an answer, and this is when my fight began.

In the process of testing they found my blood pressure to be very high. I suffered a mini stroke and had therapy for six months to regain the use and mobility of my left arm and leg.

Things went downhill fast. They could not get my blood pressure under control. Medicine after medicine, specialist after specialist, and things were not getting better. My doctor was stunned and scratching his head in disbelief as to what was wrong. He sat by my hospital bed and cried with me, and he has fought for me from day one.

I spent a year bedridden. My blood pressure fluctuated badly, and keeping my blood pressure under 180/125 proved to be a challenge for every specialist I saw.

Over the next six years I saw over two hundred doctors. My medical file grew, but no answers came. I am very lucky to have not had one doctor say to me, "There is nothing wrong." They saw it. They dealt with the symptoms, but the tests were just not showing anything.

"How could that be?" seemed to be my famous words. There has to be something wrong and something we can do about it. I went from playing kickball, advising cheerleading, running, being involved with my family, to constant pain and fatigue. My blood pressure fell upon standing, so I had dizzy spells, blackouts, weakness, with episodes that would take me to the emergency room and take weeks to recover from.

It seems my blood pressure was the center of it all. I could not take the anti-inflammatory drugs due to my blood pressure. I could not take any over-the-counter allergy medicines.

The doctors knew they had to bunch all my symptoms together and they knew they were all the result of one thing, but they mimicked so many diseases. With each new test came more puzzles and confusion.

Not only was it hard for me, but I also had to deal with watching my family suffer with me. My husband, who had always been supportive and caring, became frustrated watching me suffer. I decided to stop having seeing doctors since they never came up with any answer. I thought I had to be crazy or that it was all in my head.

One night after a very big episode, my husband took it upon himself to call my doctor and start testing again. We started again in Pittsburgh, Pennsylvania. I was armed with my heavy medical records, and a very negative attitude of *here we go again.*

However, I liked the doctor. He was very caring, funny, and determined to find an answer. I started having tests, that, believe it or not, I had never had before. After the second visit he said I had autonomic nervous system disorder, or dysautonomia. This is a failure of the autonomic nervous system, which handles everything that the body does naturally, without thinking, such as, breathing, blood pressure regulation, gastrointestinal function, and motor skills. Dysautonomia can cause blood pressure to suddenly drop, instead of rise, upon standing, which can cause dizziness, fainting, and fatigue.

However, this was not the primary cause of my health problems. I was sent to a new rheumatologist. I thought I might have mixed connective tissue disease (MCTD), but he thought I had signs of scleroderma, so he sent me to a dermatologist. The dermatologist took a skin biopsy, which showed signs of MCTD along with myositis.

My blood pressure medicine was quadrupled in hopes of regulating it. They say I may have a hard time with all the treatments for this because my blood pressure spikes very high.

They have not identified a primary disease yet, or one that stands out over any other, in the MCTD. I continue to have very bad episodes that confine me to my bed for weeks. I use a wheelchair for long excursions, and family trips. I carry a blood pressure monitor with me and a lifeline medicine, nitroglycerin. We have to know where all the hospitals are when we travel.

This diagnosis is a bittersweet one. After seven years of hell, I thought a diagnosis would come with a treatment or a cure, but that was not the case. My family struggles daily with the stress of having a sick mother and wife. We fight daily for strength, courage, hope, understanding, and love.

Recently my nine-year-old daughter started showing signs of an autoimmune disorder, and I am once again terrified. But this time I am armed with knowledge and wisdom. Will my experience become a path of knowledge to help my daughter and to keep her from struggling like I did? If so, it would have all been worth it for me.

I have a very loving husband who always tried to understand and help me with the constant pain and disabilities. I have four beautiful children who help me stay grounded and who give me the strength to go on. I have a wonderful sister who lives far away, but her daily e-mails and gifts of love and encouragement remind me to see the blessings in my everyday struggles.

I continue to have good days and bad, and very bad episodes. My symptoms include (but are not limited to) high blood pressure, seizures, muscle pain and weakness, joint swelling, vision problems, gastrointestinal and pulmonary difficulties, fibromyalgia, lumps under my skin, stiffness, and the list goes on.

If I can help prevent just one person from suffering like I have, my fight will have been worth it. God bless all of you who suffer and survive a chronic illness or who have had to see your loved ones suffer.

In ending my story I will tell you that my new nickname is *Lucky*. Lucky to have had three rare diseases in one lifetime. I like to see it as being blessed.

❖ ❖ ❖

Nathalie
Switzerland

My name is Nathalie and I am twenty-eight years old. I was diagnosed with scleroderma and lupus about six months ago. In January 2002, I arrived at the hospital with two black fingers. They had gangrene and I was very worried about having an amputation. I could not possibly imagine my life with some fingers cut off.

Since that time, five of my fingers have been partially amputated. I am even relieved about that because it was very difficult and painful to live with gangrened fingers. Now I accept my hands as they are and I can handle everything as I could before.

Let me tell you my story from the beginning. Four years ago the doctors found out that I did not have enough platelets in my blood and that it was due to the fact that I had too many antibodies. So I had to take prednisone, which is a derivative from cortisone. But as soon as I stopped this medicine, my platelets went down again, so the doctors decided to take out my spleen. After that operation, the doctors told me I might have lupus, but they gave me no more information, just that I need to have my platelets checked regularly.

I was twenty-four years old, still studying, and I wanted to enjoy life. For four years I led a happy and interesting life. Nevertheless, I had some symptoms during that time which are typically linked to lupus, such as Raynaud's phenomenon, swollen knees, hair loss, mouth ulcer, infection under some fingernails, and two big ulcers in my left leg.

Every time I talked to the doctor about these symptoms, he said to me that it was nothing worth being worried about. I sometimes complained about my extremely cold hands turning white, yellow, orange and then blue and he said it was due to stress. I told him about my infection under some fingernails and he said it would go away with time. I did not know that lupus or scleroderma were the cause of my blue hands. I now realized that I suffered a lot from this lack of information. Every time I talked to the doctor about my symptoms, I felt stupid and I thought that I was complaining about small things.

In 2001 I finished my studies and I started working as a high school geography and English teacher. In November I absolutely wanted to heal the infection under my fingernail, so I decided to change my doctor and went to see three other doctors. From then on I saw a doctor almost every week until the end of January. During January it was extremely cold. The cold was almost killing me and the infection under my fingernails hurt so much that I could not sleep at night.

It is still very painful for me to remember that period of time, because I told my doctor that I had the impression that there was no blood in my little finger any more. He said, "I am not going to give you some medicine just because you have cold hands."

Two weeks later I had to go to hospital with two black fingers. It was a terrible day for me. The doctors told me I had an incurable disease and that I had to stay in hospital for weeks.

I was very sad and angry because I had just started working and my boyfriend and I had decided to get married in March and to have a big party. Many questions were going through my head:

- Am I worth living?
- Am I going to die?
- Why should they keep me at work if I am sick?

At the beginning it was very difficult for me. I realized that my disease—lupus, scleroderma or whatever, even the doctors did not know what to call my disease—would not go away and that I have to live with it for quite a while. During my stay in the hospital I was lucky because my husband, my family and friends gave me great support.

A lot of people visited me every day during the five weeks! But I had black fingers and they had never seen that before, so I had to face many reactions. Some people cried (even some men!), some were very surprised, some did not show anything. What I hated most was to hear the sentence: "Oh, poor girl, you are really unlucky."

It was also very difficult for my parents to accept that I had an incurable disease. After many long discussions, now my relationship with them is even better than it was before.

Concerning my husband, we married on March twenty-ninth, but we did not have a big party. He has always accepted me as I am, and he has helped me through very difficult times.

In the hospital, a psychiatrist helped me a lot, especially in accepting my disease. I could simply talk about my things that bothered me, and we practiced hypnosis. I imagined my blood flowing better in my veins and reaching my fingers. We also tried to fight my pain with hypnosis, and it worked.

Since May, I have been leading a normal life again. Of course, after I came out of the hospital I had to tell my story several times. But now that my fingers have healed well, I think people rarely notice my strange hands anymore. Today I like my hands because I can use them as before, and that is more important than how they look.

I think I will be able to live quite a normal life. Of course, I will have to see the doctors regularly, and I have to stay in the hospital every six weeks for three days (but I can go home for the night). I am a bit worried about that, because I do not know how I am going to reconcile this with my work, but I am sure there is a solution.

The disease has not attacked my internal organs. My lung capacity is reduced, but my kidneys work well. I still can do everything I did before, so I have decided to make the best out of this and to be in good spirits.

Sometimes I am angry because I think I might not have acted early enough with my fingers, but then I remember that I went to the doctor all the time.

If my doctor had taken my symptoms more seriously, earlier, maybe my gangrene would have been prevented, so I am hoping that my story will help someone else avoid a similar situation.

I really want to have children now. The doctors told me that I have to wait at least one year and then we will see. The day I can hold my little baby in my arms will be a real victory for me!

Robin E.
Georgia, USA

I do not know if I can describe what I am going through, because it changes every week, if not every day.

It started with swelling and pain of my feet, hands, and legs, which I thought was arthritis. I have had fatigue so bad that I never thought I would make it through the day.

Now my hands and fingers are raw and sore. I have to use them every day with my work. I put lotions on them and antibiotic ointments and sometimes sleep with gloves on. Yet I still have nothing but ulcers, and it is like all the skin is peeling off my fingers, making them raw.

I have been told I have scleroderma by a specialist, but I have no idea what type yet because more tests are being run. The last time I went to him, he told me one of the tests showed lupus, too.

I am almost forty-two and I have been healthy almost my entire life. My symptoms just began in January 2002, so everything seems to be happening fast.

Susan McIvor
Canada

I am a fifty-two year old woman living in mid-Canada. In 1993, I was a single parent of two teenagers when I developed extreme fatigue, aching joints, and Raynaud's.

I was first diagnosed with lupus by my family doctor, and then with CREST by a rheumatologist. My symptoms remained fairly stagnant for about six years.

Then I started having extreme muscle and joint pain, very swollen hands, esophageal problems, and constant nausea. My Raynaud's had also worsened, making it more challenging to live here, since our winter temperatures are as cold as forty degrees below.

I limped through the next few years, with ongoing fatigue that would stop me in my tracks. I think fatigue has been the worst problem for me to deal with.

I have continued to work a full time job, although I am not sure how much longer I will manage it, since I do not have any energy left at the end of the workday. I was recently diagnosed with Hashimoto's hypothyroidism, and I am hoping that treatment for that will reduce my fatigue.

My loved ones and my family and children have been supportive. Especially, my daughter has been a brick, and I enjoy my three wonderful little granddaughters.

My former family doctor—who I recently dismissed—told me I should just stop complaining and get on with things, because everyone has aches and pains. He would not follow my rheumatologist's directions regarding medications, and refused to follow up with regular testing.

I have a fabulous new doctor now, so I have been able to put those dark times behind me, and enjoy the sunshine.

◆✧◆

PART 4

International

CHAPTER 9

Español (Spanish)

Francisco
Morfea
Bogota, Colombia

This story was translated from Spanish to English by Edwin Lamoli-Torres, who is a retired professor from the University of Puerto Rico at Mayaguez. The English version of this story is in Chapter 6.

Bien, hace 15 dias me diagnosticaron esclerodermia morfea. Note la presencia de la enfermedad cuando comenzaron a salir unas manchas en mi tronco con apariencia inicial de moretones; luego la piel se fue poniendo dura y con apariencia quebradzia, como cicatrizada.

Tengo manchas de variados tamaa'os en la espalda, el muslo, el brazo, la mano, el pie, y en la cintura, todas en el hemisferio izquierdo.

Me siento muy afligido a causa del diagnostico, pues mi dermatologo ha dicho que la enfermedad es cronica y que su tratamiento va a durar aa'os, por ahora me han prescrito colchicina y una emulsion para aplicarme sobre las manchas.

Si alguien puede indicarme algo mas sobre el tema, os quedare muy agradecido. Y si de algun modo puedo yo colaborar en algo pues no duden en escribirme.

CHAPTER 10

Italiano (Italian)

Chiara
Italia

This story was translated from Italian to English by Kevin Howell. He is a Clinical Scientist for Professor Black at the Royal Free Hospital in London. The English version of this story is in Chapter 5.

Sono Chiara, ho 19 anni e da 14 anni sono affetta da sclerodermia localizzada (morphea). In tutti questi anni non ho fatto altro che "balzare" da un ospedale all'altro! Sono stata ad un ospedale dove mi hanno "torturato" con infiltrazioni di cortisone.

Finalmente, dopo quasi 4 anni di cure, arriva la mia ancora di salvezza, l'ospedale De Marchi di Milano. Qui i medici sono riusciti a fermare la malattia! Una grande vittoria dopo tanti anni di sofferenza!

Maria Clemente
Italia

This story was translated from Italian to English by Kevin Howell. He is a Clinical Scientist for Professor Black at the Royal Free Hospital in London. The English version of this story is in Chapter 6.

La malattia di cui sono affetta mi è stata diagnosticata nel 1998, anche se i primi accertamenti sono stati eseguiti circa due anni prima, a seguito delle manifestazioni della stessa, in uno dei migliori ospedali dermatologici italiani. Io penso, anche sulla base di informazioni raccolte, che l'inizio della mia malattia sia strettamente legato ad un lungo periodo di insonnia e conseguente stress emotivo, in seguito alla presenza di un dolore all'emicostato legato all'osteoporosi.

All'inizio è apparsa una macchia perlacea delle dimensioni di una moneta al centro della schiena, tra le scapole; la lesione si presentava con un bordo rossastro di circa 5 mm. In seguito la macchia si è estesa fino a raggiungere un'estensione di circa 7 cm di diametro con indurimento e depressione della zona di pelle interessata. Altre piccole macchie sono comparse successivamente in altre zone (avambracci e gambe), questa volta scure e con una leggera depressione. Dai vari esami, come la biopsia cutanea con relativo esame istologico, la manometria esofagea e la valutazione della funzionalità polmonare, è risultata solo una lieve insufficienza respiratoria (con la possibilità, tuttavia, che tale quadro sia l'esito di un episodio di polmonite in età giovanile). Non risultava però un coinvolgimento a livello sistemico. Penso che il danno maggiore sia a carico della vista, manifestatosi con un repentino peggioramento funzionale dell'occhio, in concomitanza allo sviluppo della malattia.

Vorrei, se possibile, il vostro parere su un'eventuale evoluzione della malattia ed anche dei consigli su come eventualmente curare la mia forma. Grazie.

❖❖❖

Roberta
Italia

Ciao, mi presento, sono una ragazza di 31 anni affetta da questa patologia da circa 7 anni e sono in cura al centro IDI di Roma. Per una settimana ogni mese mi reco in questo centro, dove vengo sottoposta a terapia vasodilatatrice (con alprostadil), l'unico sistema finora che (secondo loro) può, in qualche modo, arrestare la lenta progressione di questa malattia.

Non mi ha mai spaventato tanto l'idea di esserne affetta, ma una cosa ora mi preoccupa e mi rattrista: sono sposata da 2 anni e avrei desiderio di un figlio, ma ho paura per lui e soprattutto per me. I medici, non è che mi sconsigliano del tutto la gravidanza, ma mi avvertono sempre delle conseguenze (nove mesi senza cura sono tanti!). Vorrei sapere se c'è qualcuno nella mia situazione che può darmi validi consigli ed incoraggiamenti. Aggiungo che la malattia si è fermata alle mani con ulcere e pelle dura ma non ha interessato nessun organo interno.

CHAPTER 11

Polski (Polish)

Dorota
Twardzina Linijna (Coup de Sabre)
Poland

Moja historia z twardziną zaczęła się 15 lat temu i do dzisiaj (kiedy trafiłam na strony serwisu o sklerodermii) nie zdawałam sobie sprawy z tego, jak poważną chorobą może być twardzina oraz jak wielkie mam szczęście, że moja choroba przybrała tak łagodną postać. Zresztą dopiero z internetu dowiedziałam się czym tak naprawdę jest skleroderma, ile osób na nią choruje i że na świecie są książki, grupy wsparcia, poradnie itd. W Polsce chyba niestety nadal niewiele się w tym kierunku dzieje i dlatego też zdecydowałam się umieścić tu także i moją historię.

W wieku 16 lat, w wakacje, po powrocie z rocznego pobytu Syrii (piszę o tym, bo być może ma to jakieś znaczenie...) zauważyłam na czole, u nasady włosów jasną plamę - wyglądało to tak jakby podczas opalania coś zasłaniało fragment skóry, który w wyniku tego pozostał blady. Zresztą tak to sobie na początku tłumaczyłam.

Opalenizna zniknęła, a zmiana pozostała i miałam wrażenie, że się powiększa - o ile pamiętam skóra była w tym miejscu biała i błyszcząca, rodzina się śmiała, że ktoś przyłożył mi palec do czoła i zostawił znak - tak to wyglądało. W końcu poszłam do dermatologa (w mieście stołecznym Warszawa, a jakże) – lekarz stwierdził, że na pewno mam to od urodzenia tylko wcześniej "mamusia nie zauważyła" - żenujące... "Znamię" się powiększało, "weszło" we włosy i włosy na fragmencie skóry wypadły.

Zaniepokojona tym wszystkim Mama znalazła dojście "po znajomości" do pani dermatolog. I tak trafiłam do Instytutu Dermatologii. Pani dermatolog nie zbagatelizowała mojej przypadłości i rozpoznała ją jako sklerodermię, dla pewności zaprowadziła mnie jeszcze do pani profesor (niestety nie pamiętam w ogóle nazwisk) dla potwierdzenia diagnozy. Dość dziwnie się czułam, kiedy panie zaczęły nagle przy mnie rozmawiać po angielsku (tylko, ze ja znam angielski) i mówić, że nie umrę. Ale potraktowałam to jako drobne dziwactwo pani profesor.

I mówiły jeszcze "en coup de sabre"—sprawdziłam w słow-niku: cięcie szablą. Leczenie było następujące: trzy serie penicyliny po 30 zastrzyków (jeden dziennie), witamina e i piascledine (sprowadzana z wielkim trudem z Francji - na szczęście mój Tata miał jakieś możli-wości.).

Potem już tylko piascledina i witaminy. Robiono mi co jakiś czas badania kontrolne - chronaksję czuciową (to pamiętam, bo miły pan mi mówił, że jestem "milionerką") i jakieś z krwi - generalnie nic strasznego się nie działo. Zmiana na czole "zeszła" prawie do nosa i "weszła" jakieś 5 cm we włosy, z tym że najszersza (ok. 1,5 cm) jest w górnym odcinku, a niżej to już tylko kreseczka. Dotykając palcem wyczuwa się jakiś brak - tak jakby pod skórą była od razu kość. Po leczeniu "sklercia" przybrała kolor brązowawy, a włosy częściowo odrosły. Piascledinę przyjmowałam seriami jeszcze przez dwa czy trzy lata, potem zarzuciłam leczenie i kontrole - nic się nie działo.

I tak przez kolejne dziesięć lat z hakiem żyłam ze sklerodermią nie przejmując się nią zbytnio, czasem tylko ktoś z nowych znajomych pytał czy w dzieciństwie byłam strasznym łobuzem, skoro tak sobie rozcięłam czoło. No i wtedy miałam okazję opowiadać o dziwnej i nieznanej nikomu chorobie - sklerodermi. Czasem "sklercia" się uaktywniała - dostawała sinej obwódki, ale ponieważ nie "schodziła" niżej nic z nią nie robiłam. Zresztą miałam wrażenie, że uaktywnia się w momentach stresowych mojego życia. Mniej więcj w tym samym okresie pojawiły się mi na plecach dwie pręgi w poprzek kręgosłupa, które początkowo brałam za odciśnięcie od zapięcia stanika. Zostały jednak na zawsze, wyglądają troszkę jak rozstępy, mają ok. 10 cm długości, czasem są prawie niewidoczne, czasem bardziej wyraźne i swędzą - myślę, że to również może być sklerodermia.

Jak widać moja sklerodermia nie przeszkadzała mi zbytnio wżyciu i mam nadzieję, że tak pozostanie. Chociaż ostatnio znowu się uaktywniła (sina obwódka, wyraźniej ją widać) i mam wrażenie, że obok niej skóra jest bardziej błyszcząca i bielsza. To mnie zanie-pokoiło i dlatego zaczęłam szukać w internecie wiadomości na ten temat. Zamierzam wybrać się z nią do lekarza. Mieszkam teraz na Dolnym Śląsku i mam nadzieję, że i tu znajdę kompetentnych lekarzy - zwłaszcza, że sądząc po informacjach, które dziasiaj znalazłam, przez te 15 lat wiedza na temat tej choroby zdecydowanie się zwiększyła, no i zapewne piascledinę (jeśli nadal się ją stosuje) teraz można łatwiej zdobyć. Na dzień dzisiejszy tak się przedstawia moja historia. Zoba-czymy co będzie dalej.

◆ ❖ ◆

Eliza
Teściowa, Morfea
Poland

This story was translated from Polish to English by Dr. Roy Smith and Dr. Magdalena Dziadzio. The English translation can be found in Chapter 2.

Serdecznie witam. Mam na imię Eliza i właściwie nie chodzi o mnie tylko o moją teściową.

Trzy lata temu na udzie zrobiła się jej ranka; teściowa podejrzewała, że skaleczyła się i od tego ma strupek. Zmiana skórna po jakimś czasie zaczęła się to powiększać, poszła więc do dermatologa, który pobrał jej wycinek z tego miejsca.

Niestety nie postawił jednoznacznej diagnozy i zaczął ją leczyć na chybił trafił; zastosował nawet kurację sterydami, która nie odniosła jednak żadnego skutku. Pomimo przyjmowania przeróżnych tabletek i smarowania tego miejsca maściami nie było poprawy i nowe ranki pojawiły się pod piersią i pod pachą.

Teściowa zrezygnowała z tego lekarza i przeniosła się do innego, który również pobrał wycinek i rozpoznał chorobę: "sklerodermia." Pan doktor stwierdził, że jest to choroba nieuleczalna, ale niezbyt groźna i trzeba nauczyć się z nią żyć i na tym zakończył leczenie.

W międzyczasie bardzo spuchła jej noga na wysokości kostki. Teściowa poszła więc do reumatologa, który po wynikach stwierdził, że jest to zapalenie naczyń chłonnych i może to być powiązane ze sklerodermią.

Reumatolog poinformował nas, że sklerodermia nie jest wcale chorobą niegroźną, że może mieć związek z chorobą żołądka, na którą teściowa leczy się już od kilku lat jak również z astmą. W końcu dodał, że sklerodermia może zatakowac całe ciało łącznie z kośćmi i organami wewnętrznymi.

Kogo słuchać? Kto ma rację? Gdzie szukać pomocy?

Na zakończenie dodam tylko, że teściowa ma 58 lat, w swoim życiu miała kilka operacji i przyjęła niezliczone ilości lekarstw (nie jest lekomanką).

Dziękuję za zainteresowanie.

❖ ❖ ❖

Ewa
Syn Albert, Linijna (Coup de Sabre)
Poland

This story was translated from Polish to English by Dr. Roy Smith and Dr. Magdalena Dziadzio. The English translation can be found in Chapter 5.

Moja historia z Twardziną zaczęła się cztery i pół roku temu, w 1997 roku w listopadzie. Wtedy urodził się nam synek Albert, wyczekiwane i ukochane dziecko. Na początku, tzn. przez pierwszy miesiąc jego obecności na świecie, nasze życie to była bajka, niewyobrażalne szczęście i radość, że urodził się nam piękny i silny chłopczyk ważący 4000g i 57cm długi. Według skali Apgar miał on przy urodzeniu 8 punktów, ale co tam. Sina nóżka i coś w jąderkach to nic i faktycznie jąderka doszły do normy po tygodniu. Nóżka nie. W miesiąc po urodzeniu Albercik został skierowany do szpitala z powodu zachłystowego zapalenia płuc, ciągle krztusił się pokarmem, ale doskonale przybierał na wadze i w miesiąc przybrał 2 kilogramy. I wtedy się skończyło i zaczęło się.

Obawy taty Alberta, że jego nóżka jest chudsza od drugiej, były przez lekarzy komentowane, że "taka to jego uroda," a to, że jej skóra jest jak marmur, "wymyślanie dzieciakowi choroby na siłę." Po tygodniu w szpitalu ja i tata Alberta byliśmy wyczerpani i biliśmy się z uczuciami, co się dzieje i dlaczego lekarze tak się zachowują. Żyliśmy tak przez rok i nic się nie działo. Albert siadał w wieku trzech miesięcy, chodził jak miał dziewięć miesięcy, a kiedy skończył rok, był już wprawnym chodziarzem, tylko nie rozmawiał i często chorował. Poza tym wszystko układało się jak najlepiej, z wyjątkiem podróży do Centrum Zdrowia Dziecka i niezliczonych badań, w celu dowiedzenia się, dlaczego jego jedna noga jest sucha, szara (właściwie marmurkowa), odrobinę zniekształcona i chuda, a druga różowa, miękka i pulchna jak u bobasa. Kiedy Albert skończył rok i trzy miesiące zauważyłam, że dziwnie się zachowuje, a kiedy powiedziałam o jego zachowaniu lekarzowi skwitował on, że "wygląda mu to na padaczkę, ale żeby się nie martwić." Ja nie mogłam przestać myśleć o tej opinii i pojechałam z dzieckiem na prywatną wizytę do neurologa dziecięcego do Olsztyna. Tam, po usłyszeniu moich słów, pani doktor chwyciła za słuchawkę w swoim gabinecie i zorganizowała mu badanie EEG. I okazało się, że mój instynkt nie kłamie i Albert jest chory na epilepsję. Na całe szczęście zauważyłam pierwsze objawy i skończyło się na dwóch napadach. Teraz bierze leki i jest dobrze.

W międzyczasie na chorej nóżce pojawiła się plama, a właściwie znamię (1,5cm na 2cm); było ono dziwne, bo w czerwonej "ramce" i takie grube, szorstkie i swędzące. Poszłam do dermatologa, który przepisał maść Elocon. Na początku była poprawa, bo zmiana nie była czerwona, ale za to bardzo piekło smarowanie, które sprawiało ból Albertowi. Dodatkowo po Eloconie Albert zaczął budzić się w nocy z krzykiem, że boli go cała noga! To było dziwne, dermatolog zmieniał maści, przepisywał różne emulsje i płyny do kąpieli i nic, a plamka rosła i rosła i ból był coraz większy.

W międzyczasie urodziła się siostra Alberta Asia, a Albert ani myślał zrezygnować z ssania piersi i ssał ją do prawie czwartego roku życia. Pewnego dnia u Asi pojawiło się dużo krostek na całym ciele. Ja i mąż już mieliśmy dość "pogoni za wiatrem" po Giżyckich przychodniach, przy okazji wizyty w Olsztynie u neurologa postanowiliśmy pójść do dermatologa. Sądziliśmy, że ma on na pewno więcej doświadczenia, niż nasza dermatolog w Giżycku. I stało się: po wejściu do gabinetu z dziećmi okazało się, że Asia ma wysypkę bo ja pewnie coś zjadłam, a kiedy poprosiłam aby lekarka wypowiedziała się na temat Alberta, ta niewiele myśląc sięgnęła po telefon i wezwała reumatologa na konsultację. Na koniec ja siedziałam i płakałam, a pani doktor wypisywała mi promesę do Warszawy, bo u Alberta stwierdzono Twardzinę. Nie wiedziałam, co to jest, ale pani doktor powiedziała: "jak się szybko uda wszystko zorganizować, to nic złego mu nie będzie, ale jest to choroba nieuleczalna, a niektóre przypadki kończą się śmiercią." To jedno zdanie sprawiło, że nie pohamowałam łez i znienawidziłam tę Twardzinę. Pojechaliśmy do Warszawy a tam pewna pani doktor zaczęła na mnie krzyczeć, że za późno i że źle, że Albert był szczepiony itd. Później na sali, kiedy zapytałam co to znaczy Twardzina usłyszałam zdanie, które było początkiem końca "znam takich, którzy z Twardziną, jak u Alberta, rodziny zakładają" a ja usłyszałam, że on umiera.

Po serii badań okazało się, że Albert ma objaw Raynauda to znaczy, ze ma jakieś "pętle w paznokciach." Zlecono mu leki i zabiegi: masaż, laser, gimnastyka, pływanie, masaże wirowe itd. Wysłano nas do domu. Po roku od wizyty w Warszawie plama, która rozrosła się do rozmiarów około 10 cm i zbladła, znikła prawie zupełnie; zostawiła po sobie dziwną bliznę i szarą owłosioną skórę. Teraz tylko jeździmy do reumatologa do Olsztyna i jest dalej wszystko dobrze z małym z wyjątkiem, że mój instynkt nie pozwala mi czuć, że już będzie dobrze do końca. Ciągle słyszę słowa tych lekarzy w głowie i zastanawiam się, co jeszcze mogę zrobić, aby mu pomóc. Teraz ma wkładkę w prawym bucie wyrównującą długość kończyn. Ja zrobiłam tę wkładkę pod całą stopą mimo, że lekarz kazał dać 1,5cm wyrównania pod piętę. Boję się każdego kaszlnięcia, czy to już się znowu zaczyna, czy to tylko grypa. Kiedy jest grzeczny, zastanawiam się dlaczego, czy już jest chory czy nie. Poza tym jest normalnym chłopcem, który szaleje i broi, kiedy tylko się da. Boi się pobierania krwi więc robimy badania co cztery-pięć miesięcy, a nie co miesiąc.lato, znowu będę używać kremu z dużym filtrem lub blokera na jedną nogę, a z małym na drugą, aby nie było widać zbyt dużej różnicy w kolorze nóg. No i znowu będzie mógł pływać dzień w dzień w jeziorze. A za dwa lata, kiedy pójdzie do szkoły, to może nikt nie zauważy na lekcjach gimnastyki, że on jest inny.

Bóle nogi nie są takie częste jak kiedyś; skóra po zabiegach lasera jest bielsza, a włosy na nodze po laserze są słabsze i jaśniejsze. Krem Lipobase powoduje, że skóra jest miękka; hulajnoga utrzymuje nogę sprawną, rower zapewnia ruchomość stawów, pływanie w wodzie sprawia mu przyjemność i usprawnia go fizycznie i teraz już jest bardzo silny. Piłka kangurka jest niezastąpiona, a najbardziej lubi, kiedy może sam sobie smarować nogę płynem z oliwką. Wtedy wynajduje kosteczki i mówi: "to są kości mojego ciała; to ciało jest twarde, a to miękkie." Ostatnio zapytał naszą znajomą, która ma sześciomiesięcznego synka: "jeżeli Maciuś też ma bolącą nogę, to ja mu dam taki krem i nie będzie go boleć."

To dla mnie coś, co sprawia, że mój synek musi nosić but ortopedyczny i coś, co powoduje, że nie jest taki, jak inni chłopcy. A dla Alberta coś naturalnego i oczywistego, na co nie zwraca uwagi. Czasem tylko na podwórku słyszę jak koledzy go pytają: "czemu masz taką nogę?" a on mówi: "bo to jest moje ciało i musi być twarde!"

Chapter 12

Русский (Russian)

Моя (Maria)

Ukraine

This story was written by Maria in English and translated back into Russian by Dr. Alexandra Balbir-Gurman. The English translation can be found in Chapter 3.

Все началось с того, что у меня стали белеть и неметь кончики пальцев при охлаждении.

Поначалу приступы длились недолго, но вскоре стали возникать даже в тепле, и длиться больше.

часа. К этому времени врачи установили диагноз синдрома Рейно. Вскоре появились утолщение кожи на лице и пальцах, множественные ранки на руках, а также воспаление суставов.

Прием Бутадиона не принес облегчения. Кроме того у меня появились изжоги и боли в животе, и лечение Бутадионом я прекратила. В последсвии у меня установили болезнь склеродермию, и я была госпитализирована в ревматологическом центре и получила лечение гепарином, дексаметазоном и вливания илопроста (простациклина). В результате лечения мне стало немного лучше: постепенно язвочки зарубцевались, но я прдолжала страдать от болей в мышцах и потеряла много в весе.

В последнее время я чувствую себя хуже из-за слабости и, одышки и сердцебиений, и болей в груди при малейшей нагрузке. Мои руки искривились и с трудом сжимаются в кулак.

Меня одолевают запоры, аппетита нет совсем и я продолжаю худеть. Приступы синдрома Рейно возникают в руках и ногах и в последнее время вновь появились признаки изязвления на пальцах. Цвет моих пальцев меняется от белого до синего. Я очень скованна и с трудом расхожусь к середине дня. Я живу в холодной стране и очень страдаю особенно зимой. Мне установили частичную инвалидность и я с трудом работаю часть дня (в школе).

К сожалению, в моем городе нет специалиста по склеродермии, а наблюдаться в специализированном центре у меня нет возможности.

Я сознаю что заочныя консультация носит ограниченный характер, но у меня нет сомнения, что специалист в данной области да и сами больные склеродермией могут помочь советом. Поэтому мне важно существование сайта по проблемам склеродермии в интернете.

Conclusion
by Shelley L. Ensz

Voices of Scleroderma has shown us the height of courage of those who have lived, and died, with scleroderma and related illnesses. We have all given our stories—as patients, caregivers, survivors, and researchers—in the hopes of making it easier for others.

The two hundred stories in this series so far have just begun to tell the saga of scleroderma, which is so vastly different in every case with its onset, severity, symptoms, course and outcome.

Not even a thousand stories would clearly expose the dire and urgent need for more scleroderma information, support, awareness, and research throughout the world.

Yet, at the same time, every single story does tell the story of scleroderma; every single story does expose the need for a cure; every single story offers its own ray of hope, its own form of support.

Have you found solace and strength in this book and courage to continue your battle with illness or caregiving? Have you wept with grief or compassion from the stories of those who are suffering, or who have died?

Have their plainly detailed struggles whisked you away to seldom visited corners of your soul, changed the way you feel about your life, your health, your loved ones, your values, and the importance of cherishing each and every moment?

Whether or not you or a loved one has scleroderma or related illnesses, if you feel warmed by compassion and stirred to action by our plight of the "disease that turns people to stone," we invite you to continue to support the cause of scleroderma in your community and throughout the world.

By joining forces together, person by person and story by story, link by link, and group by group, someday our voices of scleroderma will be heard all around the world!

Someday, there will be a cure! And it will be because we all left our footprints on the sands of time.

"Footprints, that perhaps another, sailing o'er life's solemn main, a forlorn and shipwrecked brother, seeing, shall take heart again."

◆❖◆

Glossary of Medical Terms

A

acid reflux

A burning discomfort behind the lower part of the sternum usually related to spasm of the lower end of the esophagus or of the upper part of the stomach often in association with gastroesophageal reflux. *See also: heartburn*

alopecia

Hair loss or baldness.

amputation

Removal of part or all of a body part enclosed by skin.

antibody

A special protein produced by the body's immune system that recognizes and helps fight infectious agents and other foreign substances that invade the body.

antinuclear antibodies (ANA)

Antibodies or autoantibodies that react with components and especially DNA of cell nuclei and that tend to occur frequently in connective tissue diseases (as systemic lupus erythematosus, rheumatoid arthritis, and Sjögren's syndrome).

arthritis

Inflammation of a joint. When joints are inflamed they can develop stiffness, warmth, swelling, redness and pain. There are over one hundred types of arthritis.

aspiration pneumonia

Infection of the lungs due to aspiration (the sucking in of food particles or fluids into the lungs).

autoimmune disease

An illness that occurs when the body tissues are attacked by its own immune system, such as Hashimoto's thyroiditis, polymyositis, rheumatoid arthritis, scleroderma, Sjögren's syndrome, and systemic lupus erythematosus.

B

Barrett's esophagus

Metaplasia of the lower esophagus that is characterized by replacement of squamous epithelium with columnar epithelium, occurs especially as a result of chronic gastoesophageal reflux, and is associated with an increased risk for esophageal carcinoma.[1]

biopsy

The removal and examination of the tissue, cells, or fluids from the living body.[1]

bowel disease, inflammatory

A group of chronic intestinal diseases characterized by inflammation of the bowel, such as ulcerative colitis and Crohn's disease.

C

calcinosis

An abnormal deposit of calcium salts in body tissues, as is seen in some forms of disease, including CREST, which is a form of systemic scleroderma.

carpal tunnel syndrome (CTS)

A condition caused by compression of the median nerve in the carpal tunnel and characterized especially by weakness, pain, and disturbances of sensation in the hand and fingers.

CAT scan

A scan using computerized axial tomography.[1]

collagen

An insoluble fibrous protein of vertebrates that is the chief constituent of the fibrils of connective tissue (as in skin and tendons) and of the organic substance of bones.

connective tissue disease

Any of various diseases or abnormal stats (as rheumatoid arthritis, systemic lupus erythrmatosus, polyarteritis nodosa, rheumatic fever and dermatomyositis) characterized by inflammatory or degenerative changes in connective tissue.[1]

CREST Syndrome

A limited form of systemic scleroderma.

CT scan

A scan using computerized tomography.

D

diffuse scleroderma

A form of systemic scleroderma that generally involves widespread skin involvement.

dysphagia

Difficulty swallowing[1]

E

echocardiography

The use of ultrasound to examine and measure the structure and functioning of the heart and to diagnose abnormalities and disease.[1]

eosinophilic fasciitis (Shulman's syndrome)

A disease that leads to inflammation and thickening of the skin and a lining tissue under the skin, called fascia, that covers a surface of underlying tissues.

esophageal

Of, or relating to, the esophagus (throat).

esophagram

A series of X rays of the esophagus. The X ray pictures are taken after the patient drinks a solution that coats and outlines the walls of the esophagus. Also called a barium swallow.

ESR
Abbreviation for erythrocyte sedimentation rate.

F
fainting (syncope)
To lose consciousness because of a temporary decrease in the blood supply to the brain.
fibromyalgia
Any of the group of nonarticular rheumatic disorders characterized by pain, tenderness, and stiffness of muscles and associated connective tissue structures.

G
gangrene
Local death of soft tissues due to loss of blood supply.[1]
gastroesophageal reflux
Backward flow of the gastric contents into the esophagus resulting from improper functioning of the sphincter at the lower end of the esophagus.[1]
gastrointestinal (GI)
Of, relating to, or affecting both stomach and intestine.
GERD
Abbreviation for gastroesophageal reflux disease. A highly variable chronic condition that is characterized by periodic episodes of gastroesophageal reflux usually accompanied by heartburn and that may result in histopathological changes in the esophagus.

H
heart failure
A condition in which the heart is unable to pump blood at an adequate rate or in adequate volume.
heartburn
A burning discomfort behind the lower part of the sternum usually related to spasm of the lower end in association with gastroesophageal reflux.
hernia
A protrusion of an organ or part through connective tissue or through a wall of the cavity in which it is normally enclosed.
hiatal hernia
A hernia in which an anatomical part (as the stomach) protrudes through the esophageal hiatus of the diaphragm.
high blood pressure
Hypertension; abnormally high arterial blood pressure.
hypertension
Also known as high blood pressure; abnormally high arterial blood pressure.

hypothyroidism

Deficient activity of the thyroid gland. A resultant bodily condition characterized by lowered metabolic rate and general loss of vigor.[1]

I

inflammation

A local response to cellular injury that is marked by capillary dilatation, leukocytic infiltration, redness, heat, pain, swelling, and often loss of function and that serves as a mechanism initiating the elimination of noxious agents and of damaged tissue.[1]

interferon

Any of a group of heat-stable soluble basic antiviral glycoproteins of low molecular weight that are produced usually by cells exposed to the action of a virus, sometimes to the action of another intracellular parasite (as bacterium), or experimentally to the action of some chemicals, and that include some used medically as antiviral or antineoplastic agents.[1]

interstitial cystitis (IC)

A chronic idiopathic cystitis (bladder inflammation) characterized by painful inflammation of the subepithelial connective tissue and often accompanied by Hunner's ulcer.

irritable bowel syndrome (IBS)

A chronic functional disorder of the colon that is characterized by the secretion and passage of large amounts of mucus, by constipation alternating with diarrhea, and by cramping abdominal pain.

J

juvenile scleroderma (JSD)

Any form of scleroderma that afflicts children. The localized forms of scleroderma (such as linear and morphea) are most common in children.

K-L

limited scleroderma or limited cutaneous systemic sclerosis (lcSSc)

A form of systemic scleroderma where the skin involvement is limited to the hands and/or face.

linear scleroderma

A form of localized scleroderma, a line of thickened skin that can affect the bones and muscles underneath it, thus limiting the motion of the affected joints and muscles. It most often occurs in the arms, legs, or forehead, and may occur in more than one area. It is most likely to be on just one side of the body. Linear scleroderma generally onsets in childhood, and is sometimes characterized by the failure of one arm or leg to grow as rapidly as its counterpart.

localized scleroderma

Scleroderma that affects only the skin and not the internal organs. Types of localized scleroderma include morphea and linear.

lupus
>Any of several diseases (as lupus vulgaris or systemic lupus erythematosus) characterized by skin lesions. *See also: systemic lupus erythematosus (SLE)*

lymphoma
>A usually malignant tumor of lymphoid tissue.[1]

M
migraine
>A condition that is marked by recurrent usually unilateral severe headache often accompanied by nausea and vomiting and followed by sleep, that tends to occur in more than one member of a family, and that is of uncertain origin though attacks appear to be precipitated by dilatation of intracranial blood vessels.[1]

mixed connective tissue disease (MCTD)
>A syndrome characterized by symptoms of various rheumatic diseases (as systemic lupus erythematosus, scleroderma and polymyositis) and by concentrations of antibodies to extractable nuclear antigens.

MRI
>A procedure in which magnetic resonance imaging is used.[1]

morphea scleroderma
>A form of localized scleroderma that affects only the skin, causing skin patches that may be red, brown, white or purplish in appearance.

multiple sclerosis (MS)
>A demyelinating disease marked by patches of hardened tissue in the brain or the spinal cord and associated especially with partial or complete paralysis and jerking muscle tremor.

N
neuropathy
>An abnormal and usually degenerative state of the nervous system or nerves; also a systemic condition (as muscular atrophy) that stems from a neuropathy.[1]

O
oesophagus
>Alternate spelling for esophagus.

osteoarthritis
>Arthritis of middle age characterized by degenerative and sometimes hypertrophic changes in the bone and cartilage of one or more joints and a progressive wearing down of apposing joint surfaces with consequent distortion of joint position usually without bony stiffening.[1]

P-Q
palpitations
>A rapid pulsation; an abnormally rapid beating of the heart when excited by violent exertion, strong emotion or disease.

peripheral neuropathy

A problem with the functioning of the nerves outside the spinal cord. Symptoms may include numbness, weakness, burning pain (especially at night), and loss of reflexes.

petechiae

Pinpoint flat round red spots under the skin caused by intradermal hemorrhage (bleeding into the skin).

plaque, skin

A localized abnormal patch on a body part or surface and especially on the skin.

pleurisy

Painful and difficult respiration, cough and exudation of fluid or fibrinous material into the pleural cavity.

pneumonia

An infection that occurs when fluid and cells collect in the lungs.

prostaglandin

Any of various oxygenated unsaturated cyclic fatty acids of animals that have a variety of hormone-like actions (as in controlling blood pressure or smooth muscle contraction).

pulmonary fibrosis (PF)

Scarring throughout the lungs which can be caused by many conditions, such as sarcoidosis, hypersensitivity pneumonitis, asbestosis, and certain medications.

pulmonary function test (PFT)

A test designed to measure how well the lungs are working.

pulmonary hypertension (PH)

High blood pressure in the pulmonary arteries.

PUVA

PUVA stands for psoralen and ultraviolet A (UVA) therapy in which the patient is exposed first to psoralens (drugs containing chemicals that react with ultraviolet light to cause darkening of the skin) and then to UVA light.

R

Raynaud's or Raynaud's Phenomenon or Raynaud's Disease

A vascular disorder that is marked by recurrent spasm of the capillaries and especially of the fingers and toes upon exposure to cold, that is characterized by pallor, cyanosis, and a redness in succession usually accompanied by pain, and that in severe cases progresses to local gangrene.

reflux, esophageal

A condition wherein stomach contents regurgitate or back up (reflux) into the esophagus (throat).

rheumatoid arthritis (RA)

A usually chronic disease that is considered an autoimmune disease and is characterized by pain, stiffness, inflammation, swelling, and sometimes destruction of joints.

rheumatologist

A specialist in rheumatology, a medical science dealing with rheumatic diseases, which are any of various conditions characterized by inflammation or pain in muscles, joints, or fibrous tissue. Scleroderma is considered to be a rheumatic disease.

S

sclerodactyly

Scleroderma of the fingers and toes.[1] Swelling, tightening, curling, and hardening of the fingers and/or toes, as caused by the systemic forms of scleroderma.

scleroderma

A disease of the connective tissue. There are many different types of scleroderma. Some affect only the skin, while other types also affect the internal organs. *See also: diffuse scleroderma, linear scleroderma, localized scleroderma, morphea scleroderma*, and *systemic scleroderma*.

sedimentation rate

The speed at which red blood cells settle to the bottom of a column of citrated blood measured in millimeters deposited per hour and which is used especially in diagnosing the progress of various abnormal conditions.

seizure

Uncontrolled electrical activity in the brain, which may produce a physical convulsion, minor physical signs, thought disturbances, or a combination of symptoms.

Sjögren's syndrome

A chronic inflammatory autoimmune disease that affects especially older women, that is characterized by dryness of mucous membranes especially of the eyes and mouth and by infiltration of the affected tissues by lymphocytes, and that is often associated with rheumatoid arthritis.[1]

skin plaque

A plaque is a broad, raised area on the skin. Because it is raised, it can be felt.

stem cell transplantation

The use of stem cells as a treatment for cancer or other diseases.

systemic lupus erythematosus (SLE)

An inflammatory connective tissue disease of unknown cause that occurs chiefly in women and that is characterized especially by fever, skin rash, and arthritis, often by acute hemolytic anemia, by small hemorrhages in the skin and mucous membranes, by inflammation of the pericardium, and in serious cases by involvement of the kidneys and central nervous system.[1]

systemic sclerosis (SSc)

The type of scleroderma that can cause damage to skin, blood vessels, and internal organs. Subtypes include CREST, limited and diffuse scleroderma.

T

telangiectasia

An abnormal dilatation of capillary vessels and arterioles that often forms an angioma. (Plural: telangiectasias or telangiectases.)[1] Often casually referred to by patients as *red spots* or *red dots* on the face or hands.

thyroiditis, Hashimoto's

A chronic autoimmune thyroiditis that is characterized by thyroid enlargement, thyroid fibrosis, lymphatic infiltration of thyroid tissue, and the production of antibodies which attack the thyroid and that occurs much more often in women than men and increases in frequency of occurrence with age.

titer or **titre**

The strength of a solution or the concentration of a substance in solution as determined by titration.[1]

total parenteral nutrition (TPN)

Intravenous feeding that provides a patient with fluid and essential nutrients. Also referred to as *tubal feeding*.

tracheostomy

The surgical formation of an opening into the trachea through the neck especially to allow the passage of air.[1]

U

ultrasound

A noninvasive technique involving the formation of a two-dimensional image used for the examination and measurement of internal body structures and the detection of bodily abnormalities.[1]

undifferentiated connective tissue disease (UCTD)

When a person has symptoms of various connective tissue diseases without meeting the full criteria for any one of them, it is often called undifferentiated connective tissue disease.

V-Z

ventilator

Also known as respirator. A mechanical device for maintaining artificial respiration.

vitiligo

A skin disorder manifested by smooth white spots on various parts of the body.[1]

[1] By permission. From *Merriam-Webster's Medical Dictionary* © 2002 by Merriam-Webster, Incorporated.

❖ ❖ ❖

Index

O

X

X rays 83, 85, 98, 142, 169

Y

Yale University Medical Center 169

About the Editors

Judith Thompson Devlin is Chair of the ISN Archive Development Committee and author of three published novels: *The Kiss of Judas*, *A Switch In Time* and *Mind Blindness*. She also collaborates with Shelley Ensz for the ISN's *Voices of Scleroderma* book series.

She resides in New Hampshire. She was diagnosed with CREST/systemic sclerosis in 1991 and has been on disability since then. Judith attended Dean Junior College in Franklin, Massachusetts. She holds a certificate for successful Hospice Volunteer Training and for Mediation Training.

She participated in a drug research program for scleroderma at the Boston University Medical Center with Dr. Joseph Korn as well as participated in the Scleroderma Family Registry and DNA Repository with NIH, presided over by Dr. Maureen D. Mayes.

Shelley L. Ensz is Founder and President of the nonprofit International Scleroderma Network, the Scleroderma from A to Z website, the Scleroderma Webmaster's Association, and EdinaWebDesign.com. She lives in Minnesota with her marvelous husband Gene, and their delightful Senegal parrot, Webstergirl.

The **International Scleroderma Network (ISN)** is a nonprofit organization that provides scleroderma medical and support information and works to raise awareness of scleroderma throughout the world. We also support international medical research for scleroderma through the ISN/SCTC Research Fund.

The ISN is an outgrowth of the Scleroderma from A to Z website at www.sclero.org, where the personal stories in this book were first published. Our website offers over one thousand pages of scleroderma medical and support information in eighteen languages.

Over five dozen virtual volunteers from around the world operate the ISN website, book series, online support community, medical advisory, translation services, hotline, email support, and newsletter production services. We invite you to become an ISN member, donor and/or volunteer today, and help us put an end to scleroderma!

❖

Scleroderma Resources

International Scleroderma Network (ISN)

The ISN is a nonprofit, charitable organization that offers worldwide medical, support, and awareness information for scleroderma and related illnesses.

Scleroderma Clinical Trials Consortium (SCTC)

The SCTC is a charitable, nonprofit organization dedicated to finding better treatment for scleroderma. Over 50 SCTC member institutions worldwide conduct clinical treatment trials for scleroderma, and they publish the Scleroderma Care and Research Journal. See **www.sctc-online.org**.

ISN/SCTC Research Fund

You may support international scleroderma research via the collaborative ISN/SCTC Research Fund.

ISN's Scleroderma Webmaster's Association (SWA)

The SWA features Worldwide Support Group listings and the ever-popular *Scleroderma Sites to Surf!* Get your group or website listed today!

ISN's Scleroderma from A to Z Web Site "Sclero.Org"

The ISN operates the Scleroderma from A to Z site at **www.sclero. org**, where the personal stories in this book were first published. The site offers over one thousand pages of top quality scleroderma medical and support information in many languages.

This section for use by ISN, SWA, SCTC, scleroderma, or arthritis-related groups, centers, or organizations:

◆ ❖ ◆

ISN Membership and Donation Form

The International Scleroderma Network (ISN) is a nonprofit organization. We welcome members from all countries who are interested in scleroderma or related illnesses. We also strongly encourage you to join your local or national scleroderma or arthritis associations.

❑ **Voices of Scleroderma Book Series** Please notify me when other books in this series become available for purchase.

❑ **Volunteer** I am interested in volunteering for the ISN.

❑ **Online Annual Membership** Enclosed is my donation of $25 or more (U.S. funds only) for an ISN Online Membership (in English) to receive the ISN Insider newsletter only by email.

❑ **Regular Annual Membership** Enclosed is my donation of $35 or more (U.S. funds) for an ISN Regular Membership (in English) to receive the ISN newsletter through postal mail.

❑ **Donation–For Research Only** Enclosed is my gift in the amount of $_____ (U.S. funds) for the ISN/SCTC Research Fund to support international research for scleroderma.

❑ **Donation–Nonmember, General Use** Enclosed is my gift to the ISN. You may use the funds as you see fit. I understand that a portion of my donation will go to the ISN/SCTC Research Fund. I do not want to receive the ISN newsletter or other membership benefits.

❑ **Donation–In Honor or In Memory of** Enclosed is $_____ in honor or in memory of _____.

❑ **Donation–Special** Please contact me, as I would like information about making a stock donation, in-kind, matching funds contribution, or bequest.

Your Name (first, last): _____

Address: _____

City: _____ State:_____ ZIP:_____

Country: _____ Phone:_____

Email: _____

Pay by: Total: $_____ (U.S. funds)
❑ Check   Cardholder: _____
❑ Visa   Card #: _____
❑ Mastercard   Card Expiration Date: (month/year): _____
❑ AMEX   Verification Number: On the back side of your card, there is a long number. What are the last four digits? _____

Please mail this form with payment made out to:
International Scleroderma Network
7455 France Ave So #266
Edina, MN 55435 USA

❖❖❖

7077531R0

Made in the USA
Lexington, KY
18 October 2010